Physicians in the Academic Marketplace

Recent Titles in
Contributions to the Study of Education

Between Understanding and Misunderstanding: Problems and Prospects for International Cultural Exchange
Yasushi Sugiyama, editor

Southern Cities, Southern Schools: Public Education in the Urban South
David N. Plank and Rick Ginsberg, editors

Making Schools Work for Underachieving Minority Students: Next Steps for Research, Policy, and Practice
Josie G. Bain and Joan L. Herman, editors

Foreign Teachers in China: Old Problems for a New Generation, 1979–1989
Edgar A. Porter

Effective Interventions: Applying Learning Theory to School Social Work
Evelyn Harris Ginsburg

Cognitive Education and Testing: A Methodological Approach
Eugene J. Meehan

American Presidents and Education
Maurice R. Berube

Learning to Lead: The Dynamics of the High School Principalship
Gordon A. Donaldson, Jr.

Windows on Japanese Education
Edward R. Beauchamp, editor

Integrating Study Abroad into the Undergraduate Liberal Arts Curriculum
Barbara B. Burn, editor

Managing Institutions of Higher Education into the 21st Century: Issues and Implications
Ronald R. Sims and Serbrenia J. Sims, editors

Identity and Ideology: Sociocultural Theories of Schooling
Stanley William Rothstein

Moral Education and the Liberal Arts
Michael H. Mitias, editor

PHYSICIANS IN THE ACADEMIC MARKETPLACE

DOLORES L. BURKE

Foreword by Theodore Caplow

CONTRIBUTIONS TO THE STUDY OF EDUCATION, NUMBER 53

GREENWOOD PRESS
New York • Westport, Connecticut • London

Library of Congress Cataloging-in-Publication Data

Burke, Dolores L.
Physicians in the academic marketplace / Dolores L. Burke : Foreword by Theodore Caplow
p. cm. — (Contributions to the study of education, ISSN 0196-707X ; no. 53)
Includes bibliographical references and index.
ISBN 0-313-27850-4 (alk. paper)
1. Medical colleges—United States—Faculty. I. Title. II. Series.
[DNLM: 1. Career Mobility—United States. 2. Faculty, Medical. W 19 B959p]
R745.B86 1992
610.69'52—dc20
DNLM/DLC
for Library of Congress 91-28327

British Library Cataloguing in Publication Data is available.

Library of Congress Catalog Card Number: 91-28327
ISBN: 0-313-27850-4
ISSN: 0196-707X

First published in 1992

Greenwood Press, 88 Post Road West, Westport, CT 06881
An imprint of Greenwood Publishing Group, Inc.

Printed in the United States of America

The paper used in this book complies with the Permanent Paper Standard issued by the National Information Standards Organization (Z39.48-1984).

10 9 8 7 6 5 4 3 2 1

Contents

Tables

Foreword

In this admirable book Dolores Burke explores the world of academic health centers, whose inner workings are nearly unknown to outsiders. Previous research in the sociology of academic institutions, including Burke's own study of faculty replacement in the arts and sciences departments of research universities (*A New Academic Marketplace*, Greenwood Press, 1988) showed that their complexity can be conveniently approached by interviewing the people involved in recent faculty hirings and terminations. That simple procedure is a key that unlocks many puzzles.

Universities are more complex than industrial corporations or government agencies for several reasons. Their tasks are more differentiated, and the cognitive distances between the specialists who perform those tasks are much greater. The professor of physics and the professor of French literature nominally follow the same occupation, but neither has a clear idea of what the other does. The managers of universities—presidents, provosts, deans—are unlike other managers. They cannot supervise, evaluate, or even understand the work performed by their subordinates, and there is no bottom line to tell them whether the return on investment is better in microbiology or in semiotics.

Universities are also unique in rewarding their academic employees less for the work—mostly teaching—that they are paid to do than for the work—mostly research and writing—that they undertake voluntarily. This has been the subject of pious protestation ever since the American university assumed its present form almost a century ago, but it is inherent to that form.

Multiple constituencies are another source of complexity. The modern American university must satisfy at least seven major constituencies: students, alumni, faculty, staff, administrators, research sponsors, and outside regulators—and innumerable minor ones. These constituencies have few interests in common, and their demands on the university are dramatically incongruent.

In the academic health center complexity is raised to a higher power. The basic functions of teaching and research are bifurcated into clinical and non-clinical, but clinical practice must also be viewed as a function separate from teaching and research. New constituencies appear, including patients, insurers, nurses, attending physicians, and hospital administrators. The division between undergraduate and graduate students gives way to finer gradations: students, interns, residents, and fellows. The faculty divides into tenure and non-tenure, clinical and non-clinical, teaching and non-teaching, and M.D. and Ph.D. The subspecialties and the subsubspecialties multiply.

Above all, monetary issues become salient. The academic health center is no ivory tower where scholars are given a modest stipend to pursue a life of reflective contemplation. It is a place for big investments in new technology, big deals with research sponsors, big revenues from patient care. At my own university last year, eight members of the medical faculty were paid more than the president—up to three times as much. It is not uncommon for the head of a medical subdepartment to build a new wing or establish a new clinic with funds under his sole control. Increasingly, teaching and research are supported by patient fees, and medical faculty members are judged by the income they produce. "At all ranks and levels of responsibility," writes Burke, "the new faculty member was expected to generate all or part of his or her own salary through research grants and/or patient care."

These phenomena reflect the extraordinary levels to which physician incomes in the United States have been pushed by twenty years of massive federal subsidies through Medicare, Medicaid, and the National Institutes of Health. The average American physician is better paid than a U.S. Senator and medical fees rise inexorably from year to year, defying all efforts at cost containment so far.

That situation has all sorts of favorable effects for the medical sector of the academic marketplace. Since full-time service on a medical faculty does not entail much financial sacrifice, medical schools are able to recruit and hold the best and brightest people in many fields. Since private practice offers a convenient and lucrative alternative to an academic medical career, the weeding out of unsuccessful junior faculty is almost painless. And since junior faculty are selected in easy stages, by mentors who know them well and can certify that they are both professionally competent and personally compatible, there is not much weeding to do. Senior appointments are equally particularistic—the search and selection process takes place within a network of amicable peers. These procedures contribute to the exceptional stability of medical faculties, their low turnover, and the long incumbency of department and division heads.

Moreover, the decentralization of entrepreneurship in medical faculties—down to subspecialties and subsubspecialties—and the consequent weakness of bureaucratic controls has undoubtedly contributed to the spectacular improvement of surgical and pharmacological procedures and to extraordinary recent advances in those branches of science, like immunology and human genetics, that are concentrated in medical faculties.

The more troubling aspects of the institutional pattern described by Burke have to do with the relationship of the medical faculty to the university and to the larger society. Academic health centers seem to be outgrowing the universities to which they nominally belong. Their budgets, buildings, and salaries are out of scale with the relatively modest provisions made for other faculties; their sheer size inhibits intellectual or even sociable interaction with colleagues in other faculties; their ability to generate income, and the intricate modalities by which they do it, make them virtually independent of university oversight and control. As in intercollegiate athletics, another financially autonomous activity, the university often lacks the authority to influence what is done in its name.

In relation to the larger society, the very features that make the medical faculty so effective for technical purposes—narrow specialization, authoritarian management, the emphasis on expertise and compatibility, the priority of research, the need to generate income—limit its involvement with broader issues. The problems of the American health care system—excessive cost, inadequate coverage, the scanting of preventive medicine, overtreatment, excessive paperwork, and the various facets of the malpractice problem—are seldom studied in medical faculties; they do not belong to any recognized specialty, and the expression of innovative opinions on such matters is regarded as unprofessional. The effective isolation of academic physicians from national health care issues is one of the many interesting discoveries that await the attentive reader in this fine book.

Theodore Caplow

Acknowledgments

I am grateful to many people who assisted in this research. Chief among them were the medical academicians who responded to my questions—300 faculty members at six major medical schools who were willing to share with me their experiences and observations on faculty mobility. The courtesy and cooperation given by these busy professionals reinforced my enthusiasm throughout the project. Gratitude is also due to the administrators who smoothed my way through a maze of hospital corridors from coast to coast.

I thank Sydney Halpern for her early encouragement, and colleagues Fred Brown, Burton Clark, David Dill, William Donelan, Duncan MacRae, Reece McGee, David Webster, and Robert Winfree for information and criticism along the way. Thanks also to David Riesman for putting me in touch with Thomas Stossel, who in turn furnished useful information. I owe special thanks to James Bentley, Charles Killian, and Brooke Whiting at the Association of American Medical Colleges for their help; and to Joseph Greenfield, Chairman of the Department of Medicine at Duke University Medical Center, and his division chiefs—Robert Bast, James Crapo, Vincent Dennis, Edward Holmes, Allen Roses, and Wendell Rosse—for their assistance in field testing my interview instrument.

I am particularly indebted to William G. Anlyan, then Chancellor for Health Affairs; Joel Fleishman, Senior Vice President; and Charles E. Putman, then Vice President for Research Policy and Administration, of Duke University, who provided financial support for my field research and moral support as well for this project. And thanks to my staff assistant at Duke, Joan Shipman, for her help in preparing the interview data, and the reference staffs of the Duke University and Medical Center Libraries, for ferreting out elusive papers and data.

Finally, my gratitude to family and friends who, during my absences on field research trips and while the book was emerging from the word processor, performed a myriad of thoughtful and helpful acts.

Chapter 1

Background

> Professional school locales that represent and train directly for an outside occupation now bulk large in the academic profession, despite the widespread tendency to shunt them to one side in research analyses as well as in common conceptions of the university and the academic profession. . . . Medicine is at the cutting edge of changes in the professoriate.
>
> Burton R. Clark

This book is about the medical professoriate. In particular, it is about medical faculty mobility—the movement of physicians into and out of academic positions—providing insights into the organization of academic medicine within U.S. universities. The book is based on the experience of a number of medical faculty members with the recruitment, selection, and leave-taking of faculty members, sometimes including themselves. The purpose of the book is threefold: (1) To report on the phenomenon of medical faculty perpetuation; (2) to add a dimension of information about professional school faculty to the mainstream higher education literature; and (3) to encourage further investigation.

It is odd that the medical faculty is neglected in the literature, given the size and influence of a medical school in a university. The medical school may account for half or more of a research university's budget and contain more full-time faculty members in one department of internal medicine than are counted in the entire humanities division of a college of arts and sciences. Historically, too, medicine has played an important role in the development of higher education—from its place as one of the higher faculties around which the medieval university was structured to its twentieth-century leadership in scientific research.

To be sure, the medical school is more complex than the liberal arts component (or the other professional schools) of the university through its direct involvement in the health care delivery system. The school of medicine is the only part of the university that engages in on-the-job training as part of the day-to-day curriculum; the teaching hospital, with real patients, is the place where the fledgling doctor's understandings are crafted and skills are honed. It is the place where knowledge gained in long hours spent in the library and the laboratory is *applied*—prior to graduation as an M.D. and, more important, in graduate and postgraduate medical education. The medical school faculty relies in many ways on the hospital, and so finds itself caught up in all of the policy and financial issues of health care, apart from its academic mission.

Still, the medical school is essentially an academic organization not unlike the rest of the campus. The structure of a medical school is departmental, with chairmen heading departments. Chairmen report to deans and deans to provosts or vice presidents in the usual academic hierarchy. Medical faculty members participate in faculty senates and university committees, if the medical school shares the undergraduate campus location, or they adopt a similar but separate governance structure if it does not. Promotion and tenure are points of tension in the medical academic career, as they are in the arts and sciences; criteria for promotion and tenure decisions are comparable to the arts and sciences, with a heavy emphasis on research. Medical faculty members teach and advise students, conduct research, write papers and books, attend meetings of professional societies—they engage in all of the activities normally associated with the academic life.

Of course, this was not always the case. Until this century, medical education in America was the province of practitioners. It is generally agreed that the first full-time faculty members in the clinical sciences were appointed at Johns Hopkins University School of Medicine between 1905 and 1910, but "voluntary" teachers whose primary activity was private practice continued to dominate the faculties in many medical schools as late as the 1950s. Today, on the threshold of a new century, the world of medicine has changed in both evolutionary and revolutionary ways, particularly as medical research in the clinical sciences has focused more strongly on molecular biology. Now heavily dependent on a full-time faculty and with a well-developed academic research base, the medical schools are experiencing the same kinds of concerns about future staffing—the perpetuation of the faculty—that are being raised in their sister colleges of arts and sciences.

These concerns attracted my interest as an outgrowth of a study I had published in 1988 of faculty mobility processes in the arts and sciences colleges of research universities, which was a replication of an earlier study with that parameter (Caplow and McGee, 1958). Now, drawing on the wisdom of Caplow and McGee's observation that the process by which a faculty maintains its immortality in replacing its members is central to the understanding of an academic institution, I decided to follow the example of the earlier study to explore staffing processes in the medical school.

When I began writing about arts and sciences faculty, I had found a sizeable body of literature dealing with aspects of faculty mobility in the arts and sciences. This is not the case with professional schools. Much of the background material for this study has been gleaned from work on the medical profession that might include references to or implications for academic medicine. That material has been supplemented by data and analyses from the Association of American Medical Colleges and from medical professional journals, but the coverage is not comprehensive. Generally, the information provided in the following pages falls into two categories: (1) treatment of the development of medical schools within the university and (2) specific mobility data from broad studies of faculty personnel issues prepared from AAMC records and limited studies of faculty personnel issues within certain medical specialties.

THE UNIVERSITY MEDICAL SCHOOL

In the beginning, there was Abraham Flexner, who in 1910 published his Carnegie-funded study, *Medical Education in the United States and Canada*. Flexner's report was wide-ranging, covering all 155 American medical schools then in existence, and highly critical, recommending that several be closed. There were at the time three types of medical school in the West: the clinical model that had grown out of the hospital, in effect an apprenticeship for the student; the university model in Germany and Scandinavia that was branching out into experimental science; and the proprietary model that existed only in the United States. The university model of a medical school was already gaining some acceptance in the United States, much as had the German research university in its transplantation to Johns Hopkins University late in the nineteenth century. Flexner said, "We have repeatedly urged that the proper place for a medical school is within a university . . . " (p. 140); his goal has been effectively realized: In 1990, of the 126 medical schools in the United States, only fourteen were free-standing, that is, not affiliated with a university.

Flexner's investigation essentially dealt with the organization of medical education—curriculum, laboratory sciences, clinics, and research institutes, and he recommended that the organization be built on full-time faculty members. Further, he stated an ideal for medical departmental organization: "All are [would be] university departments, busy in advancing knowledge as well as in training doctors" (p. 151). Seventy-five years later, historian Charles Vevier (1987) edited the papers of a conference commemorating the anniversary of the Flexner report, wherein leading medical academicians discussed such current topics as the "dual" faculty involved in both research and teaching or patient care and the need to continue to nurture medical research within the environs of a university.

It is true, as many medical educators at the turn of the century declared, that the proprietary form of medical school was on the way out and that the change to an academic focus was already occurring; nevertheless, it seems likely that the Flexner report gave the process a strong push and that Flexner's recommendation that clinical departments be staffed with full-time faculties (though disputed at the time) was influential in twentieth-century medical school organization.

An example of a school where the process of change was well under way prior to Flexner's efforts was Harvard, where President Eliot had instituted reforms in the 1870s (Shattuck and Bremer, 1930). Harvard Medical School had only a nominal connection with Harvard University before the Eliot presidency, and the standards were low. There were few college graduates among the medical students; the students bought tickets from faculty members to courses of lectures, much as one would do for a concert series; and the experience was capped by three years of study with a practitioner whom the faculty did not need to know. Eliot forced the shift from proprietary to university school (paying part-time salaries), raised admission standards for students and qualifications for faculty members, and began, in fact, reaching outside Boston for professors in the 1880s. Specialization, which had grown out of the scientific advances of the nineteenth century, had come to Harvard; by the time Flexner's report was published, Harvard Medical School offered specializations in dermatology, ophthalmology, hygiene, laryngology, gynecology, otology, histology and embryology, orthopedics, pediatrics, and neurology. Further, the objective of the medical school was articulated in academic terms:

> To insure that the instruction given to students shall keep pace with the ever-advancing science of medicine, it is essential that the teachers keep constantly abreast of the times in their chosen fields; better still if they themselves are pioneers. Thus the second function of a medical school is to foster research and to train men to carry on investigation. (p. 589)

Neither Eliot nor Flexner envisioned the form that the university medical school would eventually take—the academic medical center (although Johns Hopkins' medical school was designed around its hospital). I borrowed the following data from Clark's (1987) vignette, "A Pentagon of Modern Medicine," in describing the UCLA Center for the Health Sciences (p. 43): The medical center contains an 800-bed hospital and several specialized clinics. It fills 35 acres of the university campus and in the last 25 years has quadrupled in size to a $110 million, 2,400,000 square foot, 10-story structure with about 20 miles of corridors. In 1980 the medical center had operating costs of $130 million against gross revenues of $132 million. The scientific enterprise of the Center's doctors and researchers brought in grants of more than $130 million.

This kind of enterprise generated, as Clark noted, "an intensity of activity not to be imagined in humanities departments" (p. 42) and quite naturally created tension within the university organization. In the 1960s, two influential private foundations created committees to examine the role and responsibilities of this ever-burgeoning animal, the academic medical center. The Josiah Macy Jr. Foundation's *Report of the Commission for the Study of the Academic Medical Center* (1970) emphasized that it was important for the medical center to be an integral part of the university. And in personnel terms, the report stressed the need for faculty participation in policy development, chairmanships of a specified term (rather than "for life," as many were constituted), and orderly peer-controlled procedures for awarding promotion and tenure. The Carnegie Commission's *Higher Education and the Nation's Health* (1970), reflecting a more external outlook, suggested that the university should encourage the academic medical center to cooperate in developing better systems of health care delivery. Various means were to be employed to do so, among them a kind of cross-fertilization in faculty resources—

increasing the use of economists, administration specialists, and behavioral scientists in the health care delivery system. In other words, the foundation committees were saying that the medical center should honor its role as a university component, but the university should recognize its role in health care. In addition, the committees saw problems in the management of human resources within the organizations and made suggestions for their joint endeavor.

In both of the 1970 reports, the medical school had been subsumed in that larger entity, the medical center, which included one or more wholly owned or affiliated teaching hospitals. The hospital was a source of conflict and complexity not only for the larger university organization but for medicine itself, as different opinions were voiced within medical academia. For example, Lewis and Sheps (1983) made a case for the academic world's responsibility to fulfill legitimate social demands—in this case, improved health care delivery. The authors characterized the medical faculty in this way: "The medical faculty . . . is made up of groups and individuals with distinctive interests and commitments, whose strength is a function of their relative prestige and the amount of money available to them" (p. 137). The prestige and money to which they referred were seen as barriers to the proper fulfillment of responsibilities, causing neglect of problems less interesting (or less prestigious) to the medical researcher. Lewis and Sheps would encourage a health services organization that would tilt academic medicine toward service, with research based on social problems.

One might draw an analogy between the Lewis and Sheps proposal and a pharmaceutical firm's research agenda—marketing analysis in the latter case and societal needs analysis in the former. The Lewis and Sheps view may be a simplistic one that does not take into account the manner in which the nation's medical research agenda is shaped by a peculiar combination of funding preferences, political pressures, and scientific curiosity. Nevertheless, it serves to illustrate the differences of opinion within academic medicine as to the proper function of the university medical school and its faculty.

The university medical school is beset by structural ambiguity—those pressures and expectations experienced at the intersection of two social structures for which the institution has different meanings (Light, 1983). There is a continuing tension between the need to provide patient care and the need to advance medical knowledge. Yet the medical school is inextricably intertwined with the university's research mission. That research mission was articulated and established during the first four decades of the twentieth century (Geiger, 1986), and the newly acquired medical schools were instrumental in defining the new research university organization. Geiger said, "In no single area was the rise of university research so swift and dramatic as in the medical schools" (p. 88). The medical schools also effected a change in the financing of higher education. The research mission was expensive; the universities needed enormous amounts of capital to support extensive facility and faculty development. But at the beginning of the century, private foundations were not supporting higher education. After Flexner's report was published, both Rockefeller's General Education Board and the Carnegie Corporation made substantial grants to improve medical education, thus beginning the practice of giving to universities.

As in the rise of research and financial support, the medical school led the way in the expansion of higher education after World War II. Full-time medical faculty positions increased by 51 percent between 1940 and 1950 and then more than doubled from 4,212 in 1950 to 11,319 in 1960 (Starr, 1982). This medical school expansion occurred largely as a result of government policy reflected in National Institutes of Health funding and Veterans Administration hospital affiliations. Concurrently, specialization was intensifying and new subspecialties were being formed, in much the same way that subfields were proliferating in the arts and sciences disciplines. Board certification in a specialty became increasingly important. Starr noted that during World War II, higher military rank was given to physicians with board certification; the status thus given to specialization was strengthened in the following years.

Specialization had a positive effect on the development of a professional ethos among the medical faculty. Halpern (1988) pointed out, in her excellent and unique study of the pediatrics specialty, that the independent pediatrics departments of the early twentieth century changed the way in which pediatricians thought about themselves. Their legitimacy was enhanced through the academic medium of an ongoing developing knowledge base. Before that time, hospital affiliations were the source of prestige for pediatricians; the medical elites had controlled hospital appointments, awarding the plums according to the position of the supplicant in the local medical hierarchy. When academic leaders usurped this power, hospital appointments came to be based on teaching and research—a fundamental change. Thus, the medical school replaced the hospital as the key institution in pediatric careers.

The influence of the hospital in graduate and postgraduate medical education (the hospital residency and possibly fellowship following M.D. training, that is, the site of specialist training) is less clearly defined and has sparked a considerable amount of controversy over the years. Flexner had considered residency training unnecessary and referred to graduate medical education as an "undergraduate repair shop" (Stevens, 1971, 1978). In Flexner's day there were only five such programs associated with universities, but after World War I the numbers mushroomed, and by 1930 about 95 percent of medical graduates were going on to residency training. Today the number is virtually 100 percent. But the graduate training has always been fragmented and largely undirected, in an academic sense. Residents are paid by the hospital and tend to identify with the hospital: A medical faculty member will say that she completed her residency at New York Hospital, not at Cornell. Residencies are frequently a reflection of hospital staffing and teaching interests rather than either academic needs for specialized research or society's demand for physicians. Attention had been paid by organizations like the Commonwealth Fund, which tackled the problems of apportioning and paying for graduate medical education in a 1985 report. Still, the question of the extent to which graduate medical education should be a university responsibility remains unresolved.

It would appear that graduate medical education is important to the university medical school because it is the source of new faculty members, as is the graduate school for arts and sciences a source for new faculty members. Also, in the medical school setting, the selection processes at work in the residency are precursors of, or in some cases substitutes for, faculty selection processes. Bosk (1979), in his participant–observer study of the surgical services at a teaching hospital, gave special attention to the training of medical students and residents. Of particular interest here is his treatment of the selection of residents who would continue through the last three years of the five-year program. Bosk stressed the gatekeeping function of the faculty who made the selection decision and the rite of passage undergone by the successful resident, who then became a junior colleague. The resident thus has the benefit of a kind of professional seasoning to which the liberal arts graduate student does not have access. There is another point of departure here: It would not be uncommon for the resident, after completing his program, to be appointed to the faculty of the school where he had trained, whereas that would rarely happen in a liberal arts department. So, essentially, many "appointment" decisions in a medical school are actually made at points of resident selection—initial acceptance, continuance, or appointment as chief resident. And how are these determinations made? The threshold criterion is technical skill, but normative standards then become paramount. As Bosk said, a resident is accepted into the ranks because the faculty members feel "that 'he's our kind of person' or 'he's our people' . . . the phrases serve as a benediction to mark the passage of a subordinate from one whose trustworthiness and skill are always open to question to one who is accepted as a group member" (p. 164). The future faculty member comes from this group of trusted subordinates, with his or her choice of academic medicine influenced by the socialization process of the residency. But the loose academic character of graduate medical education remains a part of the hospital–patient care or medical school–academics balancing act of the academic medical center that has not been adequately addressed.

A major reason for the difficulty in addressing the academic situation of graduate medical education is the financial dependence of the medical school on the hospital. Besides paying for graduate medical education, the hospital provides facilities and equipment and may provide faculty salary support. Within the context of the university, the medical school is either wholly or to a large extent self-supporting. Within the medical school, each clinical science department generates its own operating funds from research and patient income. Within the department, faculty members are recruited with the expectation that they will make appropriate contributions to the effort. Indeed, the faculty member's salary is directly affected by his or her ability to generate the income to cover it, and in today's academic medical center, the predominant source of such income is patient care (Halpern, 1987; Jones et al., 1985; Smith et al., 1987).

This patient-care income is frequently generated through a form of group practice known as a faculty practice plan, in which the full-time medical faculty member may participate. Administrative and financial arrangements vary among schools, but the presence of a faculty practice plan is usually a recruiting incentive. The income from such plans has become increasingly important to the medical school: As a proportion of medical school revenue, such income has risen from about 6 percent of the total in 1965 to 30 percent in 1981, and in terms of operating revenues it has risen from 3 to about 18 percent during the same period (Halpern, 1987). The faculty practice plan income is usually divided—not necessarily in equal parts—among the medical school dean, the clinical chairman, and the individual faculty member (Hilles et al., 1977). Uses of the practice income within the school also vary, but the dean frequently uses the money to support undergraduate medical education, and the clinical chairman may use some of the money to support junior faculty whose research programs are not yet established. And although there is a direct relationship between the faculty member's level of patient care activity and his or her compensation, there may be a cap applied by the school to discourage the faculty member from neglecting other aspects of the faculty job. As the influence of the faculty practice plan on the clinical department has grown, however, fears have emerged that the practice plan is assuming an identity separate from the medical center and, especially, that the academic mission is being diverted (Jones et al., 1985).

Flexner said about a full-time clinical faculty in his 1910 report: "The university hospital will be their laboratory; their salaries will protect them against the distractions of successful practice . . . " (p. 132). This has turned out to be an inaccurate prediction. Indeed, it may be that the university medical school has moved full circle, from a concern about individual commercialism associated with the proprietary medical schools of the nineteenth century to a concern about corporate commercialism connected with the academic medical center of the twentieth century.

But in the meantime, the full-time medical faculty has developed an academic professionalism adapted to university norms and is cognizant of faculty mobility factors not otherwise relevant to the practice of medicine.

FACULTY MOBILITY DATA AND ISSUES

The following discussion of medical faculty mobility data derives from two sources: First, faculty mobility has attracted the interest of medical specialists who have designed, conducted, and reported the results of surveys within their particular specialties. Second, an important source of mobility data are analyses conducted by the staff of the Association of American Medical Colleges, which has existed since 1890 as a central information repository for American medical schools. Two of their well maintained data bases were particularly relevant to this study: the Faculty Roster System and the Institutional Profile System. The Faculty Roster System began in 1966 as an annual survey of individual faculty member characteristics, including such items as academic rank, specialty and board certification, research training, and employment history. The Institutional Profile System contains data, in some cases dating back to 1961, on institutional revenues and expenditures, enrollment, faculty, and curriculum.

These combined sources of data bases and independent surveys have furnished material on specific elements and issues of faculty mobility.

Career Choice

At the outset, a framing issue for a consideration of medical faculty mobility is career choice. Unlike the graduate student in the arts and sciences, the typical student enters a professional school intending to practice the profession. The academic career choice rarely occurs prior to matriculation, and usually not for several years thereafter. For the medical student, the options vary according to specialty and subspecialty, but overall, the choice of academic medicine will be made by a small minority: In 1988 there were 612,000 physicians (M.D.s) in the United States, of whom 40,136 were full-time faculty members. Career choice is, of course, affected by many factors, but Funkenstein's (1978) study of medical students' career choices dramatically displayed the influence of societal factors outside the control of the medical school, such as economic incentives and ideology. Funkenstein divided medicine into "Eras" and showed the prevalent values and attraction of academic medicine in each. During the Specialty Era of the 1950s, professional competence in practice was highly valued, and only 18 percent of the student sample opted for academic medicine. But during the ensuing Scientific Era (1959–1968), when research became the dominant value, 50 percent of the students wanted academic careers. In the next two periods—Student Activism (1969–1970) and its aftermath, the Doldrums (1971–1974)—delivery of medical care became the most important concern and student interest in academia dropped to 27 percent.

That level appeared to prevail for some time; a survey of medical school graduates in 1983 indicated that about 25 percent were interested in academic medicine (Swanson, 1984). But there may be a considerable degree of differentiation among specialties and subspecialties that affects the academic career decision. There are some fields for which the academic medical center provides the only feasible environment, and others for which private practice is an appropriate setting. For example, radiologists are close to the norm at 21 percent (Hillman et al., 1989a), but cardiologists opt for academia at a much higher rate, in one study as high as 82 percent (Pritchett et al., 1986).

What are the characteristics associated with the choice of academic medicine? As one might expect, a good MCAT science subscore and an investigative interest are high-ranking positive factors, as well as the type of medical school attended and the presence of a role model on the faculty. Rather surprising—especially considering research results on arts and sciences faculty to the contrary—is the finding that factors that are *not* significant include the type of residency program and socioeconomic status (Weil and Schleiter, 1981). Negative influences might include the opinions of faculty members of other clinical departments and of nonmedical peers—You want to be a *psychiatrist*? (Zimny and Sata, 1986).

When is the decision made to enter academic medicine? According to one group of faculty members in internal medicine, 45 percent decided during medical school and 34 percent after medical school, with 21 percent saying that they decided before medical school (Davis and Kelley, 1982). Again, this may reflect differentiation among subspecialties.

There is another category of physician who needs to be considered here—the seasoned private practitioner who chooses to return to full-time academic medicine, at some financial sacrifice. In that case, the motivation is Maslow's self-actualization (i.e., maximizing one's professional potential). The benefits are the status of academic affiliation, the participation in what is seen as an exciting team that in effect defines the profession, and above all, the opportunity to work with the "incredibly bright, questioning, and energetic residents" in the academic department (Worrell et al., 1989).

Supply and Demand

A consideration of the market*place* requires some assessment of the market. Like other professional schools, in most fields the medical school is in a seller's market, where the demand for faculty members is likely to exceed the supply. According to some indicators, even this market is tightening. One report projected a need through 1990, at zero growth levels, for approximately 2,500 new faculty members per year, while the proportion of physicians choosing academic medicine was declining (National Research Council, 1981). Surveys conducted in two specialties, pathology and obstetrics and gynecology, have also indicated shortfalls. In pathology, a comparison of residents planning to enter academic medicine and anticipated faculty vacancies showed that only 50 percent of the positions could be filled (Smith et al., 1985). In obstetrics and gynecology, departments reported a 32 percent increase in need and a 65 percent decrease in the resident pool for academic positions (Pearse et al., 1987). A third source presented a problem of a subspecialty: Postfellowship experience is an established qualification for a junior faculty position in pediatric rheumatology, and so simply looking at numbers of finishing fellowships and numbers of expected vacancies does not give a clear picture of the subspecialty's ability to meet its staffing needs (Lehman et al., 1989). Much of the data are not disaggregated, and it may well be that some or many specialties and subspecialties are not facing the implied shortage, or that staffing needs have been exaggerated to improve departmental positions, but no opposing opinions have appeared in the literature.

Demographics and Mobility Characteristics

The stratification and comparative size of the medical faculty is important to considerations of mobility, as are mobility motivators. As might be expected, the full-time faculty continued the growth reported earlier, with an increase in the M.D. faculty from a total of 16,000 in 1972 to 32,000 in 1985. During this period of growth, however, mobility decreased, with new appointments dropping from a level of 14,500 in 1972 to 7,500 in 1985 and terminations of all types decreasing from 8,400 in 1972 to 5,500 in 1985. While activity lessened, of course, the mean age of the faculty rose slightly, from 42.8 in 1972 to 44.8 in 1985 (Jolly, 1986). Comparable figures from pathology indicated a mean age of 45.2, with 33 percent of the faculty under age 40 and 8 percent over age 60 (Smith et al., 1987).

The faculty were distributed among clinical science departments that might be quite large but also quite junior, and somewhat inbred, that is, using one's own graduates on the faculty (McShane, 1977). At the time of McShane's analysis of AAMC data, clinical science faculty members ranged up to 700 in an institution, with a mean of 286 (distributed among about twelve departments of unequal size in a typical school). Almost 50 percent of the clinical science faculty were below the rank of associate professor, and about 12 percent were the school's own graduates.

The more junior faculty members, besides being the most numerous, were unsurprisingly the most highly mobile. In one study over a ten-year period, the degree of faculty mobility took the form of a perfect bell-shaped curve: 19.5 percent of faculty fell in a highly mobile group (changing jobs four times or more), 19.4 percent in a highly stable group (still at the original institution at the end of ten years), and 61.2 percent in an average mobility group (Anderson and Larson, 1975b). The highly mobile faculty members, who were usually in the lower, untenured ranks, had less responsibility in their jobs and less postdoctoral training. Also in this study, as has been found in several arts and sciences studies, faculty salary was not a significant factor in mobility.

Mobility as a function of junior status was confirmed by two studies that considered the effect of retirement on faculty demand. In the first, where retirement (and death) were studied as actual causes of mobility, a very low incidence was found, having little effect on mobility (National Research Council, 1981). A second study was concerned with the possible consequences of the elimination of mandatory retirement, and they also found minimal effect (Friedman, 1989).

An explanation of junior faculty mobility that quickly comes to mind is failure to attain promotion and tenure, which is thought to be a mobility motivator that may be particularly troublesome for a more practice-oriented specialty or individual. Yet a survey of family medicine departments and programs—surely a practice-oriented specialty—showed that although quality of research and publications was the most important criterion for promotion and tenure, faculty members *were* being tenured. Many units were finding that development of a research agenda did not require abandoning a primary care and teaching quality commitment (Holloway et al., 1989). With similar results, a study at Johns Hopkins found a widespread perception that it was more difficult to be promoted in a clinical (nontenure) track, but in fact there were no significant differences in the probability of promotion or age of promotion to associate or full professor between the two tracks (Batshaw et al., 1988).

The widely held notion that the medical academic profession loses a large proportion of its members to private practice has not been supported in the literature; a study in the 1970s showed a loss to private practice of only 7 percent of the medical faculty (Anderson and Larson, 1975a). When faculty members move from one academic job to another, the differentiation among medical schools comes into play, and the movement of faculty is comparable to patterns identified in the arts and sciences. The types of institutions between which medical faculty move are quite similar, that is, given groupings according to the school's emphasis, faculty members move within one of the groups rather than between groups (Sherman and Bryll, 1982). Generally, faculty members at a school matriculating proportionally more students with an interest in primary care specialties would move to another school with a large enrollment of students preferring primary care; faculty members of a research-intensive academic medical center would move to another research-oriented institution. A contrast to arts and sciences patterns of mobility is shown in the phenomenon of inbreeding—virtually a taboo in colleges of arts and sciences, but present in significant numbers in all medical schools. Inbreeding is somewhat higher, at 31 percent of the faculty, in the schools emphasizing primary care, but not much lower, at 25 percent, in the most research-oriented group.

Differentiation within the Clinical Department

Medical schools may share the classic higher education condition of differentiation among institutions, specialties (disciplines), and subspecialties, but there is a spreading concern about a new type of differentiation within the clinical department itself. The new differentiation—alarming to some—mirrors a split between clinical investigation and basic research in clinical science. The split has occurred as a result of three factors: (1) the changing nature of research in clinical science, shifting from a disease-oriented focus using human material, to the basic investigation in enzymes, lipids, etc., that has been made possible by advances in molecular biology; (2) the expansion of clinical departments, with an increasing dependence on patient care income, that resulted in the appointment of fewer physician-scientists to the faculty and created a need for the appointment of basic scientists to sustain the department's research activity; and (3) insufficient research training for physicians in their medical school and residency experience (Herman and Singer, 1986).

The change has been chronicled in a report based on the National Institutes of Health's data (Wyngaarden, 1979). Postdoctoral traineeships over a ten-year period had dropped for M.D.s and M.D.-Ph.D.s from 3,000 to 1,500 but increased for Ph.D.s from 550 to 1,500. The same trends were present for postdoctoral fellowships—M.D.s and M.D.-Ph.D.s down from 900 to 400; Ph.D.s up from 1,050 to 1,600—and research career development awards—M.D.s and M.D.-Ph.D.s from 60 to 50; Ph.D.s from 100 to 150. As for the proportion of new principal investigators, M.D.s dropped from 40 to 28 percent of the total and M.D.-Ph.D.s from 45 to 35 percent, but the Ph.D. share rose from 50 to 70 percent. The report's conclusion expressed a strong sentiment within clinical science: "The physician-scientist has a very special role both in posing relevant medical questions and in applying new knowledge to the investigation of disease and the teaching of students. These roles cannot be adequately filled by Ph.D.-scientists, however seminal and essential their contributions may be" (p. 1259).

Indeed, a less than sanguine view of the future held that the division could not be altered, and that although advances in science would still be taught, academic medicine would be more concerned with ideas about practical matters such as health care delivery rather than "exciting scientific ideas" (Gill, 1984). But with the increasing presence of the basic researcher in the clinical science department, there has been some urging along the lines of "join them if you can't beat them." The rationale is that it is difficult to be a part-time researcher in basic science, and a physician–scientist cannot stay at the forefront of the new science and still care for patients adequately. Two possibilities have been presented: informal physician interaction with basic scientists (Kinder, 1989) and formal medical research teams, including both M.D.s and Ph.D.s (Littlefield, 1984).

A question related to differentiation might be, who actually does the research? An examination of departments of internal medicine across institutions recorded research activity matching the research training reported above: Publication records showed that 35 percent of the M.D.s were involved in research, 55 percent of the M.D.–Ph.D.s, and 84 percent of the Ph.D.s (Beaty et al., 1986). Training was cited as an important factor in a survey of physicians in four specialties who had published in major medical journals, with 87 percent having had the benefit of two or more years in a fellowship (Neinstein and MacKenzie, 1989). And productivity across the faculty may be quite uneven. In one medical school (a less research-oriented type) during a three-year period, 25 percent of a medical school faculty authored no papers, and the 10 percent of the faculty who published the most were responsible for 40 percent of all papers published (Ellwein et al., 1989). As for the research hierarchy, the highest producers came from the specialties of (in rank order) pathology, surgery, radiology, pediatrics, and internal medicine; lowest were family practice, anesthesiology, and psychiatry. Career stage is also apparently a factor. In a radiology sample, average publication peaked at 2.2 papers per year in the second decade after training (Hillman et al., 1989b); this peak of productivity agrees roughly with Jolly's (1986) findings across specialties.

Faculty Qualifications

Although there have been no empirical studies of medical faculty recruiting that would reveal the qualifications sought in a faculty member, there are some entertaining (and informative) narratives about the process—such as a description of recruiting assistant professors as "netting small fish" and recruiting senior people as "fishing for swordfish in the Gulf Stream" (Graham, 1986) or the characterization of the recruiting process as a "mating game" (Petersdorf, 1978a). Perceptions of qualifications were plumbed in a comparison of faculty and resident attitudes at one school (a less research-oriented type), and there was agreement that the most important qualification of a faculty member was effective teaching, followed by good interpersonal skills, being well read, having private practice experience, and board certification (Crawford and Ramsey, 1984). A survey in pathology elicited the views of chairmen that research experience and specialty expertise were important (Smith et al., 1985). Perhaps the most ambitious cataloging of the general qualifications was this: general mastery of a body of knowledge of generic specialty (e.g., pediatrics) and detailed mastery of a subspecialization (e.g., pediatric cardiology); diligence in maintaining mastery as new knowledge develops; intellectual capacity to contribute to that knowledge; motivation, ability, and skills to impart knowledge to students at all levels; and the capacity and desire to use knowledge and abilities to further the goals of the university (Schofield, 1984). Of course, this superperson must also have the ability to generate income.

The need to generate patient care income to support the clinical department has created further tension with the university arts and sciences colleges, as medical schools have moved to appoint increasing numbers of faculty members who are not on a tenure track—a practice that arts and sciences faculty members view as a threat to the tenure system. At one school, the number of nontenure track faculty members rose from 55, or 9 percent of the total faculty, in 1977 to 207, or 26 percent, in 1982, with the largest concentrations in the hospital-based specialties of anesthesia and radiology (Parris and Stemmler, 1984). The criteria for the full-time track do not differ greatly from that of the tenure track appointment, with an expectation of such attributes as documented teaching performance, specialty certification, participating membership in professional organizations, and contributions to the literature. The difference in appointment would lie primarily in the allocation of "protected time" for research, and the consequent research emphasis in the faculty member's professional responsibilities.

The preceding pages give a summary of what can be learned from the literature about medical faculty mobility and the organizational environment in which it takes place. The history of university medical schools, as we know them, is recent. Although nominal connections with universities have existed since the 1700s, the medical school as an academic unit of the university is largely a twentieth-century organization—one that has been in the forefront of postwar expansion and emphasis on research in higher education. That organization has faced the typical professional school tension of structural ambiguity, with the atypical complication of direct involvement in health care delivery in America. Owing to such involvement, and dependence, some decades after specialization became the norm, the academic character of residency training is still in question, and faculty practice looms large on the scene as a necessity (financial) and a threat (academic).

As to specific mobility factors, the literature is less satisfying. The choice of an academic career, critical to sustaining the faculty, is treated in the aggregate, but information about the individual decision, and possible organizational impact on the decision, is difficult to locate. There is no current work on supply and demand across specialties in the clinical sciences. Only anecdotal information is available on recruitment and selection of medical faculty. Differences between subspecialties are not sufficiently covered in the independent studies by specialists, nor is there disaggregation in the broader studies. Generally, as is the case throughout higher education research, the researcher is hampered by a lack of data standardization; for example, it is sometimes not clear whether numbers refer only to full-time faculty or to full-time and part-time faculty.

Even so, what we know, admittedly incomplete, leads to questions about what we would like to know. What are the elements of individual decisions to attend medical school, to specialize in a certain area, and to enter academic medicine—and are there patterns of choice discernible to the academic medical organization? What is the demographic state of academic medicine; in which specialties or subspecialties do faculty members perceive staffing problems? How is faculty recruitment carried out in the clinical sciences; what are the criteria for selection; who in the organization makes the selection decisions? What are mobility motivators—why do medical faculty members leave their organizations and where do they go when they do so? What is the incidence of mobility in medical academia?

How does the environment affect medical faculty mobility? Do academic physicians make mobility decisions based on environmental factors? What is the effect of institutional policies, such as promotion and tenure, inclusion in faculty practice plans, and research requirements?

This book will attempt to provide some answers—drawn from the people who should know. The book is based on interviews conducted with 300 faculty members in six major medical schools over a period of six months in late 1988 and early 1989. The faculty members, representing all academic ranks and clinical specialties and with varying degrees of administrative responsibility, commented extensively on decisions to enter academic medicine, to take a specific faculty position, to change jobs. Their views constitute the major portion of the book, in chapters 2 through 5.

Chapter 2 provides an introduction to the marketplace, investigating the internal and external environment of the academic medical organization. Chapter 3 examines the medical faculty recruitment process, exploring such matters as the organizational justification for a faculty position, the criteria established for identifying and screening candidates, and the conduct of a search. Chapter 4 deals with questions of choice in the perpetuation of the faculty—of individual and organizational decisions and circumstances connected with joining the organization. Chapter 5 carries the consideration of choice to leaving the organization.

And finally, chapter 6 summarizes the study findings on faculty mobility in the context of academic medicine with thoughts for the future.

The stage is set. The players take their places.

Chapter 2

Introduction to the Marketplace

> The disciplines in a medical school are so remarkably intertwined. Anesthesia here is very exciting—we are involved in liver transplants and heart transplants, major trauma programs. These can't be done independently. There is this sort of strange, almost socialistic environment that exists within an academic environment.
>
> Professor of Anesthesia

> The department funding here is diversified: NIH, EPA, private industry. So that if one source breaks down altogether, it doesn't leave us high and dry.
>
> Professor of Medicine

The medical academician is a Janus-figure, very much a part of the internal environment of the medical school but highly aware of the external environment as well. It is the necessity of this dual awareness that places the medical faculty member at Professor Clark's "cutting edge of changes in the professoriate." The context of medical faculty mobility contains elements of the academic and the nonacademic even within the medical school.

This introductory chapter will present various environmental factors remarked on by the medical faculty members who were interviewed for this book. Their comments covered a broad spectrum of influences, among them the effects of specialization, the continuing emphasis on research countered by the need to produce clinical income, organizational relationships, and perceptions of the labor market. The treatment of these subjects provides a framework for the discussions of joining and leaving the medical academic organization in the ensuing chapters.

MARKET CONDITIONS

Market theory in higher education holds that academia differs from the classic labor market structure on two major dimensions. First, in higher education employers or employees are not interchangeable as they are in, for example, elementary schools or the computer industry, owing to differentiation by institutional mission. Second, the academic market is stratified by field, so that there is really no "academic profession." Academics, creating knowledge through research, have become increasingly specialized, resulting in groups of experts that make up a differential market.

Medical schools fit the higher education model but with an additional constraint: They compete directly with nonacademic organizations and self-employment situations for their faculties. Although almost everyone who earns a Ph.D. will join a work organization of some kind, the M.D. may remain independent. As a consequence, the medical schools operate in a tight labor market, unlike the condition that has prevailed in colleges of arts and sciences (although that market is showing signs of change precipitated by demographic pressures).

Department heads in all of the medical schools visited expressed concern about maintaining faculty levels. Though there was reference to national health policy as a possibly mitigating factor, some respondents thought that restrictions on the private physician's income in the foreseeable future would make academic jobs more appealing. Further expansion was also questioned; an assistant professor of surgery said, "I don't see anything in medicine growing like it has in the past." Still, there were numerous supply problems noted.

Pathology and radiology, especially, seemed to have large-scale shortages, and a variety of individual and collective strategies were communicated by chairmen of these specialties; a sampling follows:

> It's a very tight market and that's a recent development. We [professional association in pathology] have started a plan to subsidize research nationally with a heavily endowed program for residents, with the emphasis on academics.

> The academic market is very tight. There are 400 jobs out there right now. The research programs turn out about five to six hundred people a year and there are a thousand jobs in private practice. I am trying to increase the number of people going into pathology. I addressed the sophomore class in the medical school just yesterday.
>
> As a group we are trying to stimulate more academic endeavor. We have created a [training] program that is two years radiology, then a full year of research, and then two more years. We decided they needed two years so that they would think like radiologists and then they would need a couple of years to get ready for the boards. But we put the year of research in the middle.

Stratification within specialties posed special problems within an already difficult market. Uneven development of a new field, causing shortages, contributed to the stratification problem. These were comments from pediatricians and an obstetrician about their specialties:

> At the time of the major growth in medical schools, the expansion in the 1960s was evenly paced to faculty members. We got into trouble in the 1970s and are still there now, with not enough people coming through the academic training programs to satisfy some subspecialties.
>
> This is a growth area—hematology oncology—and it is hard to find people. In pediatrics generally, academicians are highly sought.
>
> There is a tightening up in some subspecialties: nephrology, metabolism genetics, child development. Generally, too, we have stiff competition from the nonacademic sector.
>
> There are more jobs than people. This subspecialty [high risk obstetrics] is the hardest to fill, and also hard to fill is oncology—there are not enough trainee slots. In high risk obstetrics, 20 percent of the training positions are vacant.

The facet of the training problem that seemed particularly critical in the primary care specialties was the need to encourage the resident's interest in academic medicine. A professor of pediatrics elaborated on the continuing problems related to training:

> The academic job market is extremely tight. Qualified people are very hard to find. It is a subspecialty issue: Pediatricians are less research oriented. Our training programs in pediatric cardiology have been focused on clinical training. There has been less interest on the part of residents in entering academic medicine. They don't know what it's like. We have no tutorial system to train academicians. We're going to have to find the very best first-year medical students and begin to cultivate them.

What these professors of medical specialties were confronting was another aspect of structural ambiguity—the career options available to an M.D. Their comments might be translated into the expression of a need for socialization into a research culture.

RESEARCH CULTURE

Research typifies the organizational culture of the contemporary research university, which is the type of institution to which medical schools are attached. The research culture is already a prominent feature in many medical schools and is becoming more prominent in others, often manifested in what respondents called a "growth in academics." For example, a more academic emphasis was observed in such diverse fields as orthopedic surgery—where a chairman said, "The field has moved away from the 'strap and buckle' era"—and pediatrics—where a chairman remarked, "We're focusing more on scholarly issues now."

The focus has shifted over the years as academic work in all fields has become narrower and more highly specialized. It has been estimated that the number of arts and sciences disciplines has doubled in the past four decades, and subfields have proliferated. By comparison, board certification in clinical specialties was fairly well established by 1950, but boards for subspecialties have multiplied since that time (see Appendix C). In both cases, expansion of knowledge—too much to be grasped completely by everybody in a discipline or specialty—has forced the compartmentalization of knowledge.

In medicine, there continues to be encouragement of greater and greater subspecialization, in which government plays a significant role. For example, a major player in the game of influencing research subspecialization is the National Institutes of Health (NIH), which in 1989 awarded $5 billion in facilities, training, and research grants to American medical schools and hospitals. NIH-funded research projects, which included topics such as "Mammalian Soluble Lectins—Properties and Functions" and "Myocardial Protein Degradation," are perhaps both a cause and an effect of subspecialization, in circular fashion. At any rate, the narrowing of research interests obviously contributes to an evolutionary trend toward stronger specialties and new subspecialties.

Examples of the strengthening of specialties were found in this study in neurology, anesthesia, and family medicine, where faculty members made these comments:

> The field has changed so much. It is a relatively young specialty, although an ancient field of medicine, but when I entered neurology in the late '40s at Yale, they had no neurologists. Now it is a small but well-defined specialty with 6,000 board certified neurologists. In 1950, there were probably none in many states. There were only a few places in the country where you could get proper training—Boston, New York, Chicago, Philadelphia.

> The specialty has persistently increased its status, so that it is attracting more medical students than it used to. When we went into it, it was a second-rate specialty, handmaid to a surgeon. Now it is broadly based, with pain management, etc., and there is good research going on in anesthesia.

> In the early 1970s, there was not much validity to family practice. It grew out of general practice and there was no academic base. Now the younger faculty members are residency trained, and it is making a difference in the departments.

And the evolution was continuing. New subspecialties would emerge as they amassed sufficient knowledge to qualify as a separate field, and eventually some might become new specialties. One emerging subfield, described by an assistant professor, was developmental pediatrics:

> Right now, in developmental pediatrics as a field, we are in turmoil because we don't have boards yet, and we are struggling to achieve a definite entity. Should we have been more closely aligned with neurology? There are variations as to where you go: What is developmental pediatrics?

The urge to subspecialize, as in the case of the closeness of developmental pediatrics to neurology, may cause some subfields in different specialties to be closer to each other than to other parts of their own specialty. Thus the "intertwining" to which the anesthetist referred carries the evolutionary trend from narrowing to widening, into the interdisciplinary nature of medicine at another level. There were numerous instances of interdisciplinarity cited in the study—the most frequently mentioned were pain management and brain science. Two chairmen in different specialties spoke of establishing basic brain science programs; one elaborated as follows:

> There is a big question today: What is the brain and who am I? For the first time we have the tools on the table to look at this question.

There is no question in the medical academic community that interdisciplinary work is important. One chairman said, "Departments are not the best way to do research." And another chairman had this recipe for success:

> People who do best in academic life are aggressive in their linkages, find people outside the department they can talk to. You can't know it all these days—it's necessary to be cooperative.

The formal programs were many, but informal interaction was also reported. One device might be a series of seminars drawing together a group of people with a common interest from different specialties and subspecialties. An assistant professor of cardiology, when we talked about subspecialization, said:

> Here we are making an effort to integrate. We have weekly conferences drawing everyone interested in the heart. It was awkward at the beginning. We were giving talks where only a handful of the group understood what we were talking about, but as the idea progressed and more people attended the meetings, we understood more and more what the others were doing. We started to get meaningful criticism from other members of the group.

Generally, the growth of research, especially molecular research, has no doubt encouraged the entry of more Ph.D.s into the clinical sciences. Concerns were raised about whether physicians were well enough trained in the newer technologies, or whether the numbers of those trained were sufficient to advance the scientific base of the specialty. A chairman said, "If you look at the research going on in the departments, it's being done by Ph.D.s." And I did not notice many attempts to integrate basic scientists and physicians in research efforts. One newly appointed chairman of anesthesia talked about proposed efforts:

> One of my jobs here is to build the research aspects of the department, and one of the most effective ways of doing that is to develop strong ties with basic scientists. Medical school does not teach you how to be a researcher.

Generally, though, Ph.D.s in clinical science departments seemed more comfortable forming professional alliances with people in the basic sciences, or in the science departments of the arts and sciences college. I did find that basic and clinical research was combined by a number of M.D.s, one of whom was especially articulate about the important role his medical training played in his basic research, "The physician's understanding of man is extremely important to [medical] research."

The increased importance of research in the organizational culture has fostered changes in the way that medical faculty members, and their departments, view themselves. At the individual level, we are more likely to find, today, medical academicians like the professor of radiology who remarked, "I consider myself an academic rather than a doctor—more aligned with those arts and sciences people that you treated in your first book." And at the departmental level, there was some reassessment taking place at schools that had been less research-oriented, as in the situation described by this chairman of surgery:

> I looked at long-term goals and decided that we were strong in the clinical arena and adequate in teaching, but we needed to grow substantially in our research orientation so that we could adapt to the future needs of the department.

These needs might take the department in a different direction in terms of staffing; one of the changes associated with the growth of a research culture was the devaluing of the voluntary faculty member—of whom there were still a large number in the schools in this study. I was surprised to find the two highest-ranked schools using heavily the services of private practitioners who brought their patients (and money) to the university's hospital in return for faculty status. One chairman of psychiatry said that he had "600 unpaid volunteer faculty members who do an incredible amount of our work," and an anesthesia chairman remarked that a third of his faculty was voluntary. At a lower-ranked school, an associate dean contributed the statistics of 728 full-time faculty (407 of them on the tenure track) and 1,235 voluntary faculty members. But it was clear that newly defined research needs were causing a re-evaluation of the volunteer physicians. In one department, a new chairman was cleaning house—one of his objectives was, "the voluntary faculty will join the clinical faculty [not tenure track but with academic responsibilities] or leave."

On the other hand, the desire for greater research activity has created financial problems for the clinical science department as the members of the department compete with a greater number of applicants for a smaller amount of research funds. Hence, there is an escalating need for other sources of income.

CLINICAL SCIENCE IN THE MEDICAL SCHOOL

As was observed in the literature, the medical school is a wholly or largely self-supporting unit of the university; however, the clinical department provides the lion's share of the medical school's revenue. The need for income that is no longer being satisfied by research dollars has in many cases forced the clinical science chair to assume the role of entrepreneur in order to keep his or her department solvent. A chairman of pathology had this to say:

> A real study would be one of the deterioration of the chairman position into entrepreneurship. The thing that's changed in pathology is that our source of funding has changed so much; to meet needs of funding you have to get your money from practitioners. Our faculty practice plan provides 50 percent of faculty salaries and I have to be constantly worrying about billing unhappy patients.

Universally, the income derived from faculty practice plans loomed large in departmental finances—although there was a perceptible whittling-away by deans who coveted a larger share of the faculty practice income for growth and development in the school. One chairman of medicine estimated that his departmental funding was 35 percent faculty practice income; a chairman of obstetrics and gynecology gave 60 percent as the proportion for his department. And a chairman of radiology cited his dean's creative accounting: a 2 percent "tax off the top" and another 10 percent or so out of net salary money.

Additional clinical income acquired through the faculty practice plan was generated by a variety of methods. One such method was by expansion of clinical programs, which might take the form of a higher volume of procedures ("7,000 deliveries" or "1,200 open-hearts") or an extension of ambulatory care. This report came from a department of medicine: "We have clinics here [the university hospital] and at the V.A. and at the state psychiatric hospital, and we are opening up satellite clinics around town."

Technological developments, sometimes combined with societal pressures, increased clinical income in some specialties. In radiology, for example, the technology of magnetic resonance imaging (MRI) was, in the words of one chairman, "revolutionizing medicine." He talked about the effect in this way: "The commercial people project that in this next year we'll do about two million MRIs and by 1991 about nine million in this country."

With respect to societal pressures, an example is the field of trauma—where a state government may become active in accrediting programs and setting up centers. An assistant professor of surgery expressed this opinion on the future of his subfield:

> Trauma is a blossoming area—very slow to develop, but over the past few years there has been gradual recognition of it by the public as a specialty, and a need for prompt trauma care. The Coasts are well served by trauma centers, and there are good systems in the North Central states, but in the Far West and the Southwest they are fairly sparse. It is a matter of politics; there are a lot of trauma centers being developed.

As that faculty member pointed out, government agencies are in turn influenced by the public, so that public awareness of the importance of trauma centers affects government priorities. In similar fashion, demographic trends in the public have another effect. Another radiologist told me that our aging population "requires more radiologic services—interventional radiology."

Beyond direct patient care, chairs were quite innovative in finding other ways to produce income. A surprising number were involved in fund-raising—apart from the efforts of the school itself. A chairman of psychiatry talked about a faculty member he had hired who "before we knew it had raised several hundred thousand dollars" for a specific program. The rationale for independent fund-raising was suggested in this comment from a chairman of orthopedic surgery:

> Increases in malpractice premiums require more patient income; that means decreasing the academic budget. Our department is 100

> years old this coming year, and we will be starting a major fund-raising campaign to try to get endowment funds to help close that gap.

Another form of external support came from industry. A chairman of radiology referred to a "sales gimmick, a form of rebate," whereby the department would buy an expensive piece of equipment and along with it get support for a certain amount of research. And a chairman of psychiatry described a "special relationship" with a pharmaceutical company in these terms: "We have a special relationship with [the company]. They invest in the department as a department, and we conduct studies for them. The investment is about $1.5 million."

Perhaps the ultimate entrepreneur was the chairman of radiology who, recognizing the financial limitations of traditional clinical income, became a small businessman:

> The bottom line is that there are only so many dollars that can be generated through the number of faculty you have. Reimbursement will be a problem, etc. I believe it will take innovative ways to deal with these problems. For example, I have put an MRI installation off-site and it is very profitable. We get the profits from both investments and the professional end.

The difficulty in balancing clinical and research needs was a constant undercurrent with the respondents in the study—much more so than any teaching versus research tensions displayed in arts and sciences departments. A clinical science department might have general research directions in which it wanted to grow, but also practical day-to-day needs in clinical coverage, and the two might not always blend. The primary care specialties, with their larger clinical loads, suffered special stress in trying to provide protected time for research. A chairman of obstetrics and gynecology said, "Patient care is the first objective, even in an academic program"; still, there was an acknowledged "need to go forward from an investigative standpoint, to advance new knowledge."

A term used frequently by clinical chairs was "critical mass"—conveying the notion that a certain number of faculty members were necessary to care for patients in order to protect some time for research. Strategies included hiring the more clinically oriented physician off the tenure track in order to free up time for differently oriented physicians to perform bench research. Examples of departments struggling with the problem were offered by two chairmen of anesthesia:

> This is a service-oriented specialty, and we've never really had enough faculty to even behave as though we had other than patient care interests.
>
> There are a certain number of anesthesia staff required to run an operating room. There should be one anesthetist for every two operating rooms; we have twenty-four operating rooms, we need at least twelve anesthesiologists. The department is also driven by academic needs—generate research, investigative work. We're going to try to do basic science research, but we need support from the medical school.

The patient care, training, and research needs of a department were summed up by a chief of thoracic surgery, as follows:

> My personal philosophy is that my division is here for three reasons: (1) to take care of patients; (2) to train cardiothoracic residents; (3) to establish a firm clinical research foundation. First you have to have clinical volume, then you've got the money to do whatever you want to do. We have a very competitive residency now. On the third aspect we're just getting geared up.

MEDICINE IN THE UNIVERSITY

The income-producing problems of academic medicine set it apart from much of the rest of the campus. Indeed, it may be largely the idea of money that creates resentment and antagonism toward the medical school from other academicians. It might be small comfort to a professor of art history to know that a professor of radiology is earning only about half what his or her income would be in private practice, when the gap between art history and radiology salaries is still sizeable. Add to this the distaste a medical school faculty member has for contributing to the support (e.g., via overhead distribution) of, say, a professor of English who "does nothing for me," as one respondent said, and the recipe for tension is complete.

And there is no question that the medical school is different from the arts and sciences college, in spite of the many ways in which it is similar. One of the most visible differences is the relationship with hospitals, especially the faculty appointment within the hospital, which appeared to be basically an economic arrangement (which included aspects of graduate and postgraduate medical education). To the faculty member, the appointment might represent individual or collective financial gain, so that the relationship was, as one professor said:

> Fairly remote on a day-to-day basis, but important as a symbol of academic goals and as a legitimacy factor for outsiders' views of the hospital (e.g., for recruitment, fund-raising, grant applications, etc.)

To the department chair, the relationship (also containing dollars) was organizationally complex. A chairman of medicine talked about his three affiliated hospitals in this way:

> We have the closest relationship with [No. 1]. Basically, it is the division of rheumatology. I have ten people there, lab space, don't have to worry about money. At [No. 2] the chairman is also vice chairman here; he is also chief of oncology. We do not have much of an oncology division here because of them, and we do have hematology, which they do not have, so our fellows move back and forth. At [No. 3] I am less involved, although the chairman is also a vice chairman here.

Medical schools, to a varying extent, may be dependent on hospitals for faculty support: "He is five-eighths V.A. FTE [full-time equivalent]," "he is paid primarily by V.A. money," and "she is really paid by Children's [Hospital]" were typical comments. Administrative arrangements are also likely to be influenced by the hospital. One chairman of pediatrics noted, "Our personnel process parallels the hospital's requirements for professional employees."

The hospitals in question have presidents and boards of trustees separate from and unaffected by those of the university parents of the medical schools. The hospitals may also exert political pressures. When questioned about faculty appointments at one of the affiliated hospitals, a chairman of neurology had this explanation:

> I think that there is some stigma regarding clinical positions and some history of political problems with [the hospital]. Although their salary schedule is higher, they feel that they are not getting their full due academically. I think that's why these people have regular appointments rather than clinical appointments.

This application of off-site faculty appointments to the tenure track, as well as the use of nontenurable clinical appointments within the medical school, has been reported as disturbing to the arts and sciences faculties who view the practice as a threat to the tenure system. Certainly, the largely self-supporting clinical science faculty members could be expected to have a perspective on tenure that might be different from that of some arts and sciences faculty members who feel they need the job security engendered by tenure. Chairmen said, "One of the worst things that has happened to universities is the tenure system," and, "Tenure is a headache." And assistant professors chimed in as follows: "Tenure is a psychological thing; it has nothing to do with anything real," and, "Tenure is a status thing." One assistant professor thought that tenure was a goal to aim for, in a sense a motivator, but "the concept doesn't mean much." An interesting observation came from a junior faculty member who had come to the United States from China: "Tenure is a socialist system; the academic setting is more like a socialist country than anything else in the States."

Views on tenure, of course, merely reflect the realities of the world in which medical academicians exist. This world is, in effect, an environment where bottom-line concerns have created a management hierarchy more corporate than academic in many respects. As I talked with junior faculty members about their work relationships, they often used the word "boss." This occurred even at the senior level, as in this quote from a division chief: "I have a number of subordinates but [the chairman] is my boss and then there are several over him." I have never heard a faculty member in the arts and sciences refer to his or her boss.

The boss in the role of the clinical department chair had both the responsibility for developing resources and authority to control those resources (in large part). Chairmanship has also been a long-term role: In this study the sixty-seven chairs (three departments were headed at the time by acting chairs) had served a total of 745 years in that position—ranging from one year to twenty-seven, with an average of eleven years. With this combination of responsibility, authority, and longevity, the chair could be expected to exert significant influence in the internal workings of the medical academic marketplace. Indeed, the clinical chairman in this study was a corporate manager, whose behavior was illustrated in this quote: "It's the chairman's decision. My mandate was to do a good job."

This introduction to the marketplace has attempted to deal briefly with several aspects of academic medicine that are believed by medical academicians to have a significant influence on their work. The market conditions, the difficulty of balancing clinical and research responsibilities, and the sources of intrauniversity tensions create an environment different from that in which the arts and sciences college functions. But the medical school is an academic institution, and the faculty members who are the participants in this study are academics, with many of the same motivations and aspirations that are found in the arts and sciences faculty. In the next three chapters, these motivations and aspirations will be explored through the processes of recruitment, selection, and separation of faculty members in the medical school.

Chapter 3

Shaping the Medical Faculty

> Recruiting is probably the most valuable thing any decent department can do. You have to have new blood, new ideas. To me, recruiting is the name of the game.
>
> Chairman of Obstetrics and Gynecology

The clinical departments in this study spent a respectable amount of effort on the recruiting game. In the one academic year covered by the study, the fifty-nine hiring departments made 207 appointments, in thirteen specialties and in all academic ranks (Table 3.1).

The recruiting, as might be expected, showed a concentration in the larger medical and surgical specialties of internal medicine, pediatrics, obstetrics and gynecology, and surgery, and also in the hospital-based specialty of radiology. The large majority of appointments were made at the junior level, and 40 percent of total appointments were not tenure eligible.

The appointments reflected what most department heads described as a typical recruiting year. There were a few departments where the activity was less than would be considered typical—such as in the department where the acting head explained, "We are in a state of waiting for a chairman," or in the department where the chairman said, "The program is growing, and we expect to recruit more in the next few years than we

Table 3.1
Appointments

	Tenured or Tenure Track				Not Tenure Track				
Specialty Group/ Specialty	Inst/ Assoc	Asst Prof	Assoc Prof	Prof	Inst/ Assoc	Asst Prof	Assoc Prof	Prof	Total
Medical									
Family Medicine		1	1			1	1		4
Internal Medicine	2	18	1	2	4	9	2	1	39
Neurology		5					1		6
Pediatrics		12	3	4		5	3	4	31
Total	2	36	5	6	4	16	6	5	80
Surgical									
Ob-Gyn	1	14			1	6	1	1	24
Ophthalmology				1				1	1
Orth Surgery		1				1			2
Otolaryngology		1	1						2
Surgery		14	1	2		9		2	28
Total	1	30	2	3	1	16	1	3	57
Behavioral									
Psychiatry		8			1	6	2		17
Total		8			1	6	2		17
Hospital-based									
Anesthesia		4		1	2	5	1		13
Pathology	1	3			1	1		2	8
Radiology		20	1	1		7	1	2	32
Total	1	27	1	2	3	13	2	4	53
All	4	101	8	11	9	51	11	12	207

did this year or last." Lack of success was identified as a cause of less recruiting activity in some instances, as in this department's case: "We had three positions that we have not been able to fill, including a section head in genetics." The reported underrepresentation was balanced by situations where recruiting was greater than usual, in "a blip for the new chairman" or in departments in "the building stage" or "a growth phase."

This chapter will explore the conditions of recruiting—the market, the need, and the process—in an effort to describe why medical faculties decide to hire, where they look for candidates, and how they go about assembling a pool of candidates from which to choose.

DECIDING TO RECRUIT

The recruiting described in the interviews extended across all specialties and included both tenure track positions and those not on a tenure track. The recruitment was categorized, in most cases, as either a replacement for someone who had left, a new position resulting from the expansion of a program, or the creation of a new program. Across specialties, the greatest recruitment activity resulted from program growth (Table 3.2), with the exception of the behavioral group, where appointments were more likely to fall in the "other" category—in this case, faculty appointments in separate agencies or hospitals that were made without substantial departmental involvement.

Program growth also accounted for most appointments regardless of tenure status or rank, except that tenured full professors were more likely to be replacements (Table 3.3).

Program growth might be explained generally as "building the department," or specifically in a number of ways. Examples of the specific references included joint expansion of a program with an affiliated hospital, often a Veterans Affairs hospital; research support for a new program, especially transplant and trauma; new divisions—thoracic surgery, pediatric anesthesia, allergy; expansion owing to new technology, such as magnetic resonance imaging (MRI); and, in a significant number of cases, expansion resulting directly from an increase in the degree or kind of patient care—group practice in the primary care fields, AIDS clinics, pain clinics, and ambulatory care.

The authorization for recruitment was quite flexible. Even where the medical campus operated under written guidelines indicating that the dean's approval was necessary in advance of recruitment, in practice the procedure for obtaining that approval was more notification than request. The chairs with whom I talked headed autonomous departments in which the decision to recruit carried their personal stamp: "I decide what we need, and I may or may not utilize other people in reaching that decision," was the comment from a chairman of obstetrics and gynecology. In a large department of medicine, the chairman said, "I make the decision about what a given division needs, what the department needs." And from a chairwoman of pediatrics came this statement: "It was my personal vision that has driven the recruitment in this department."

Table 3.2
Justification for Position, by Specialty Group

Specialty Group	Replacement	Program Growth	Other	Total
Medical	15	56	9	80
Surgical	19	28	10	57
Behavioral	4	4	9	17
Hospital-based	14	32	7	53
Total	52	120	35	207

Table 3.3
Justification for Position, by Status and Rank

Status and Rank	Replacement	Program Growth	Other	Total
Tenured or Tenure Track				
Instructor/Associate	1	3		4
Assistant Professor	20	58	23	101
Associate Professor	2	4	2	8
Professor	8	1	2	11
Total	31	66	27	124
Not Tenure Track				
Instructor/Associate	3	7		10
Assistant Professor	12	33	5	50
Associate Professor	1	9	1	11
Professor	5	5	2	12
Total	21	54	8	83
All	52	120	35	207

By far the most prevalent example of the origination of a faculty position was that in which the department chair—in concert with a division chief or an executive committee in some large departments—was heavily involved, not only making the decision to recruit but, in some cases, recruiting a specific individual. The chair's personal interest in the recruitment was evidenced in the following comments:

> The chief of the section and I discuss the need and the chief is authorized to recruit. When the group is down to a short list, I meet with each one.
>
> He was brought in to set up a research program in cell biology and the kidney. Basically, I thought he was good and so I made room.
>
> I recruited him specifically. Over a period of years I had looked at a number of people for that position. I had heard about him from somebody at McGill.

In fact, a rationale for a specific position was not always in evidence, especially in the hospital-based specialties. In those departments, recruiting was apt to be driven by a recognition of patient care demands and the knowledge that another person could be useful, as witnessed by these quotes from anesthesiology and radiology:

> We have a heavy clinical obligation, and so I'm always on the lookout for young people who are promising and may hire them even if there is not a specific slot. We need a large number of people who can work three days a week in the O.R.
>
> This was an interesting recruitment. My philosophy is different perhaps; if a truly outstanding person comes to my attention, I will recruit him and then find a place for him.

In some situations the chief of a division in a large department was instrumental in making the recruiting decision, but that did not diminish the chair's authority. In one such case, the chairman defined his role as follows:

> The division chief had 75 percent of the say. Number one, he's got the money, and it's his neck on the line. My job is to show them that the department is behind that particular effort. I view the chairmanship as a position where you carry a bag of putty around and fill holes. If a grant isn't renewed, I carry somebody over a few months. People being recruited like to know that there is some relief available.

SOURCES OF SUPPLY

Whether a decision to recruit was made or an exceptional person was noticed in some way, new faculty members came from a limited universe of residency and fellowship programs, other faculties, and private practitioners known to the department. An advantage to medical schools in a constrained market is a source of supply that differs markedly from the arts and sciences—that of the school's own residencies and fellowships. In this study, more than a third of the new M.D. appointees to junior faculty positions had completed a residency or fellowship at the institution recently or immediately prior to the appointment (Table 3.4).

The practice did not vary much among specialties, although it was used to a somewhat greater extent in the primary care fields. And, given the folk wisdom concerning the dangers of inbreeding to academic quality, one might expect that higher-ranked schools would differ in the utilization of their own graduates, but the practice did not vary by school ranking.

One chairman defended the practice of making faculty appointments from this source with the assertion, "In the medical profession, if you are a good school, you're training the best people anyway, and you can

Table 3.4
M.D. Junior Faculty Appointed from Residency or Fellowship at Hiring Institution, by Specialty Group

Specialty Group	Total Appointments	Resident or Fellow	
		Number	% of total
Schools ranked in top 19:			
Medical	32	15	46.9
Surgical	28	10	35.7
Behavioral	9	3	33.3
Hospital-based	29	10	34.5
Total	98	38	38.8
Schools ranked 20 to 50:			
Medical	19	8	42.1
Surgical	15	6	40.0
Behavioral	4	1	25.0
Hospital-based	6	2	33.3
Total	44	17	38.6
All	142	55	38.7

keep your own." Another said, "We recruit through national competition into our fellowship program and consider that good screening"; where a fellow was subsequently appointed to the faculty, the competitive selection at the fellowship point in his or her career had, in effect, substituted for a faculty selection process.

A third chairman, citing an increased use of the practice of internal recruiting, pointed to both internal and external reasons for the increase:

> We select more people from our own training programs, partly because the programs are more mature, and we have more established programs in each of the subspecialties attracting a group of trainees in both residencies and fellowships that have greater academic potential. But another reason is that recruiting from city to city is more difficult than it used to be—economic conditions, spouse factor, etc.

Along with the more important role of the internal labor market, the recruiting universe now includes more women. As enrollments of women have grown in the medical schools, the supply has moved up through the residency ranks, and that greater availability was reflected in the appointments in this study (Table 3.5).

The appointments included fifty-three women (26 percent of the total), occurring in all of the medical, behavioral, and hospital-based specialties,

Table 3.5
Appointments of Women

Specialty Group/ Specialty	Tenured or Tenure Track				Not Tenure Track				Total
	Inst/ Assoc	Asst Prof	Assoc Prof	Prof	Inst/ Assoc	Asst Prof	Assoc Prof	Prof	
Medical									
Family Medicine		1					1		2
Internal Medicine		5			2	1			8
Neurology						1			1
Pediatrics		6		2		3	1		12
Total		12		2	2	5	2		23
Surgical									
Ob-Gyn		5			1	4			10
Surgery		1				1			2
Total		6			1	5			12
Behavioral									
Psychiatry		1			1	1			3
Total		1			1	1			3
Hospital-based									
Anesthesia		2				2			4
Pathology		1			1	1			3
Radiology		6	1			1			8
Total		9	1		1	4			15
All		28	1	2	5	15	2		53

in obstetrics and gynecology and surgery, and in all academic ranks. The appointment of women followed the pattern of the total sample, with most appointments at the junior level and 41 percent not tenure eligible.

Minorities were represented as well, although in fewer numbers, and consisting primarily of Asians (Table 3.6).

The proportion of 9 percent minority appointments reflects the differentiation of supply by field and would be comparable to arts and sciences appointments in the natural sciences.

Several comments from chairs about women and minorities alluded to the variance in supply across fields:

> *Anesthesia*: The supply of women is marvelous. But I finally offered a job to a black, just yesterday, and maybe we'll get him.

> *Orthopedic Surgery*: This is a strange field, the last holdout against women. We have one resident in forty now. The field is just not attractive to women; I don't know why. And there are very, very few blacks. I wish we could attract more into the field.

Table 3.6
Appointments of Minorities

Specialty Group/ Specialty	Tenured or Tenure Track Inst/ Assoc	Asst Prof	Assoc Prof	Prof	Not Tenure Track Inst/ Assoc	Asst Prof	Assoc Prof	Prof	Total
Medical									
Family Medicine	2	1							3
Pediatrics		2						1	3
Total	2	3						1	6
Surgical									
Ob-Gyn				1					1
Ophthalmology				1					1
Surgery		2							2
Total		2		2					4
Behavioral									
Psychiatry		1				1			2
Total		1				1			2
Hospital-based									
Pathology		1			1			1	3
Radiology		2						1	3
Total		3			1			2	6
All	2	9		2	1	1		3	18

Note: Table includes two Hispanic assistant professors, appointed in Medicine and Surgery; the remaining sixteen appointments are Asians.

Pathology: There are few minorities in academic pathology. But in ten years half of pathology will be women.

Pediatrics: Individuals of ethnic or national background are rare, but with great effort we have been able to recruit three blacks in four years. Fortunately, in pediatrics there is an increasing number of women rising to the top of the academic ladder.

Radiology: We have three women professors in our department who are experts in their fields and are invited all over the world. Then we have five assistant professors who are very good. This specialty has an inordinately large number of women. It is a very collegial field and very flexible and attractive to women.

Besides an increasing use of the internal labor market and the greater availability of women, another change in the supply is a growing use of the basic scientist in the clinical science department. An indicator of the presence of basic science research in the clinical sciences is their inclusion in this study (Table 3.7).

Table 3.7
Appointments of Basic Scientists

Specialty Group	Total Appts	Ph.D.'s Appointed Junior	Senior	Total	Ph.D. % of total
Medical	80	7	4	11	13.8
Surgical	57	5	1	6	10.5
Behavioral	17	2	1	3	17.6
Hospital-based	53	9	2	11	20.8
Total	207	23	8	31	15.0

Appointments included thirty-one Ph.D.s, or 15 percent of the total. (An additional twelve appointees held the dual M.D.–Ph.D. degree or an M.D. and Ph.D. awarded separately.) The Ph.D.s were hired in all of the schools in the sample and all of the specialty groups, excluding only the specialties of anesthesia and ophthalmology. The representation of basic scientists among appointments appeared to confirm the concern expressed in the literature that the clinical investigator was an endangered species. It was felt by several respondents that the traditional training of physicians does not equip the M.D. to do the kind of research now needed, as indicated by this professor of dermatology:

> There is certainly the demise of the clinical investigator. We do not have the ability, facilities, or strength to train physicians in basic science medical investigation—that is a major problem.

In addition, respondents targeted the relationships between clinical science and basic science as a major issue in the clinical science department. But not all agreed that the M.D. was necessarily deficient in basic research expertise. As a professor of neurology pointed out: "Some of our best scientists don't have Ph.D.s. The issue is the research [that] people have done and their talent and capacity for independent thinking."

And the neurologist's viewpoint may have been validated by a newly appointed M.D.–Ph.D. who said,

> I think, looking back, if I were giving advice to somebody about what part of my training I would have omitted, it would probably have been the Ph.D. I think that you can get the equivalent training as an M.D. If my c.v. looked identical except that I did not have the Ph.D. and publication, I think I still would have gotten this job.

Regardless of the arguments, the fact in this study was a noticeable presence of basic scientists in the clinical science recruiting picture.

CONDUCTING THE SEARCH

One of the most striking features of academic hiring procedures in the arts and sciences was the time and effort that most departments expended; it took several highly skilled people a great amount of time to hire an assistant professor. Medical schools were much more practical. The conduct of the search for an assistant professor in the clinical sciences was a streamlined procedure, requiring minimal time on the part of the faculty. For example, search committees—an absolute standard in the arts and sciences—were not crucial to identifying candidates. Search committees generally functioned at a higher level in the medical world and were not concerned with junior appointments. A chairman of radiology stated, "Generally we have search committees for chiefs of divisions, but the chairman or chief would identify junior candidates."

And after such identification, the chair might proceed without involving the faculty to a great extent. I asked a chairman of anesthesiology whether or not he could act alone in recruiting a new faculty member, and he replied:

> Yes and no. The ultimate responsibility is the chairman's, but I do present all faculty applicants in detail to the executive committee of the department (the six vice chairs), and then they are also presented in a more superficial manner to the faculty overall. She didn't make a specific trip out here. I hired her after presentation to the committee.

The start of a search was routine departmental business, including the advertising of positions in professional journals, but a highly particularized recruitment took place, relying heavily on personal contacts and some direct knowledge of the candidate. (When I asked one chairman how the search had proceeded, he replied, "Very irregularly and with great difficulty.") There was very little confidence in advertising as a source of good candidates. Chairmen of pediatrics and family medicine explained the initial recruiting stages in this way:

> The division chief advertises, and then the real way we do it is to start calling people who train good fellows. We wanted someone

> who was a basic science investigator in pediatric gastroenterology, and there are a finite number of places to look.
>
> We post with affirmative action and advertise—in this case we contacted the American Academy of Family Physicians—and usually from all of those sources we get nothing. I asked the faculty going to national meetings to let the word out, and we got her name from someone in the Society of Teachers of Family Medicine.

Nor was the advertising that took place necessarily *bona fide*. It was not unusual for the motions to be gone through but the "candidate" to be preselected in what amounted to a "nonsearch," in an extreme of particularity. The nonsearch was a common occurrence, as noted in these remarks:

> He was "Outstanding Resident" the year he graduated here. We assisted him in getting a good fellowship. The protocol was: Develop a job description, advertise, interview a couple of other people in case he decided not to come.
>
> An outstanding member of the nephrology section knew about her and came to me and asked what we could do to recruit her. We did everything necessary, that is, we were careful—but we didn't look too widely.
>
> He was an outstanding trainee here who had gone off for additional training, and we succeeded in recruiting him back. We advertised, and the position was not offered until the ad had appeared and I had gotten a few responses, but there was no contest.

In another divergence from arts and sciences procedure, the speculative application was apt to be successful in the medical job market. A chairman of surgery told me about an unsolicited inquiry that landed an M.D. the job, in these circumstances:

> I was attempting to recruit a chief for the new division, but for a variety of reasons it became apparent to me that the search would have to be suspended. She wrote me a letter out of the blue asking if I had any positions open—I had been on the faculty at her school. It occurred to me that whether or not we were going to get a chief, it wouldn't hurt to have a junior person to get started—so that led

to interviews and her being hired as a member of a nonexistent division!

As for the recruitment of in-house residents or fellows, there was frequently a drifting into the faculty position, sometimes in a fairly utilitarian fashion. These were two examples from large departments of medicine:

> We needed another person, and he was a fellow here; I could hire him cheap, and I needed a "schlepper."
>
> He is one of our residents that we kept. Sometimes we have people who don't know for sure what they eventually want to do, and they are willing to fulfill the needs we have on a year by year basis.

Other recruitments of residents or fellows were more tailored to specific skills, especially in research:

> He has an extensive research background. He was highly recommended as a resident applicant and came here with a lot of support. He went through a residency and a fellowship in neuro-anesthesiology. I am always on the lookout for good neuro-anesthesiologists because we do a great deal of work in neurosurgery.
>
> She is working on several different aspects of empatic cell metabolism, liver, toxic damage. She was a fellow here and just fit into the program. She got some Liver Center funding, and the department gave her a small amount of salary, with the rest from a grant.
>
> He was in the right place at the right time. They liked what he was doing in the lab. He was largely a laboratory person but as time went on he got more involved in clinical work.

Overall, the process of deciding to fill a need followed by a search was used very little in the hiring situations in this study. One chairman referred to a "complicated story" about faculty positions, and although that degree of articulation was not presented elsewhere, and his account was incomplete with respect to specific recruitments, his narrative furnished a useful summary:

> We have a set of rules written down in the department. There are three pathways [to a faculty appointment]: (1) Self-generated—"I'm doing interesting work," "I'm in the middle of a project," "I don't want to go anywhere else," etc.; (2) also very common, a senior faculty member will designate one of his or her fellows, trying to convince the department to give a faculty title to foster that person's research career [a category not included in this study]; (3) [this method, which is] being used less and less, is what I would call the orthodox or traditional route, where a department sees a need for a new faculty position or a replacement for someone who has left and goes through the normal search process.

The normal, or traditional, search process to which he referred was used for a pronounced minority of the M.D. appointments in this study—affecting only 30 of the 142 junior appointments and 14 of the 34 senior appointments. In those cases, the search relied on a traditional academic approach where, after the department members agreed—or, more likely, after the chair or chief decided—that a particular position was required, a search committee was formed. Chairs talked about such searches in this way:

> We advertise, and then we get on the phone and we call people who might have trainees in the area. We ask at meetings; we write letters.
>
> We proceeded in traditional fashion: A formal ad, creation of a formal search committee. We sent letters to chairmen, key people in appropriate societies, selective individuals in the field. And I made innumerable phone calls.

Although there were search committees constituted for about a third of the senior appointments, such committees were usually formed by a dean in order to search for a person to fill an endowed chair, to serve as a department chair, or as the director of an important program. In another format that could apply to a senior or junior position, the chair of a medical school department collaborated with a hospital chief of service in a search, which might involve a committee composed of members selected by both.

In a senior search for a division chief in pediatrics that netted twenty candidates, this was the procedure:

There was a search committee convened headed by a pediatrics professor. There was representation from other divisions and from the medical school—the chairman of the department of human genetics, a university professor, a basic scientist, and one of the division chiefs. There is a university requirement for advertising, and then we also wrote letters to a broad group of pediatric chairmen and to specific people—for interest or recommendations—and we asked for internal recommendations. The most likely sources are internal recommendations and the chairmen.

THE RECRUITEE'S PERSPECTIVE

The new appointees themselves provided additional insights into the recruiting process. Of the 168 new faculty members interviewed, the 133 junior faculty members were successful in obtaining their jobs primarily by being there (as residents, fellows, or postdocs) or as the target of a specific recruitment effort; the thirty-five senior faculty members relocated predominantly through a school-initiated recruitment (Table 3.8).

The ineffectiveness of advertising was confirmed by the low incidence of response by new appointees. Among junior faculty members, only 6 percent of the group had responded to ads to locate their jobs, and half of those were Ph.D.s. (No senior persons responded to ads.) Even where

Table 3.8
Analysis of Recruiting, as Reported by Appointees

Appointee Status and Specialty	Response to Ad	Speculative Application	Approached by School	Internal*	Total
Junior Faculty					
Medical	4	8	13	21	46
Surgical	3	6	20	14	43
Behavioral	1	4	1	5	11
Hospital-based		5	13	15	33
Total	8	23	47	55	133
Senior Faculty					
Medical		1	15	2	18
Surgical		1	5		6
Behavioral			1	1	2
Hospital-based		3	6		9
Total		5	27	3	35
All	8	28	74	58	168

* Residents, fellows, postdocs, adjunct and voluntary faculty

an advertisement was noticed, it did not inspire action, as reported by this assistant professor and professor:

> I first saw an advertisement in the *Journal of Bone and Joint Surgery* but thought little of it until one of my staff in my fellowship asked that I consider the position and the chairman of the program called me and asked me to at least come to look at the position.
>
> I was approached as a candidate for this job as director of the division by the chair of genetics. I had also seen the ad, but I had not responded to it.

New faculty members reported using the speculative application approach rather successfully—almost 20 percent had found the method effective, as noted in these reports from three assistant professors and two professors:

> My husband had a job offer back in [this city] that was one of those you-can't-turn-down kind of things, so I called here. I talked to them at a meeting in March or April and then I came in May for a formal interview and started in October.
>
> In a sense I created it [the job]. It wasn't a posted announcement of a vacancy. I knew about the possibilities because some individuals who are in a similar line of research had called me up and invited me over to talk about sharing some patients and ideas. And at the time I thought, I'd like to come over here.
>
> My wife was being recruited here as a fellow. She was an assistant professor of pathology at Rush and then dropped out of the job market. She is an assistant professor of pathology here half-time and half-time dermatopathology fellow. I moved here and then got the best job I could.
>
> It is a long, elaborate story. Essentially, my wife was looking at a job in [this city], and I called the chairman here. Her private practice job fell through, but we decided to come anyway.
>
> I actually was down looking at a job in practice here in the city and came in and spoke with the chairman. I felt the transplant program that the private group wanted to start should be done through the university.

The appointees who had moved from residencies or fellowships to the faculty were candid about their appointments. The importance of a personal relationship was noted by this assistant professor of medicine:

> I wanted to stay in the area for personal reasons, and I had been doing work here that was reasonably productive and wanted to continue projects that I had started working on as a fellow. The section head makes decisions really on whether he likes people or doesn't like people, and I was fortunate to be liked rather than disliked.

Other new faculty members who had moved up from residency or fellowship had simply seized the opportunity:

> Well, about a year and a half into my training the general possibility was discussed with me by the section chief. He needed another clinical person, and he just raised the possibility. Then I developed certain interests in cardiology, and he could accommodate those plus an education program in which I was interested. In November someone left and it crystallized, so I stayed on.
>
> I'm not sure whether the job was open or just kind of opened up for me. I went into training without a spot to go back to and wanted to stay in pediatric neurology. They've never had a real full-time guy here, and so this seemed a good opportunity.

And the self-supporting attributes of a new faculty member were not overlooked. As one chairman had said, "We prime the pump, but we expect him to pick up 50 percent of his salary in grants." These new assistant professors recognized the importance of outside support:

> I wrote a five-year NIH grant that I got during my fellowship, and the division chief offered me to stay on here.
>
> I wanted to stay on to work with a colleague who had joined the faculty in 1985. I worked hard to get grant funding.

The limitations and serendipity of the search process were well known to the objects of the search, as was the importance of personal connections. Among those new junior faculty members in the large proportion (more than 40 percent) who were personally recruited from outside the institution, whether in a single-candidate effort or a search that generated several candidates, these comments were made:

> I received a phone call from a vascular surgeon here, the head of the section, who had gotten my name from a friend of mine who was with him in a fellowship at Northwestern. Nobody gets hired for entry level jobs without a fellowship, and there are so few vascular fellowships that it is a small network.
>
> It was really kind of a fortuitous deal in that there were two openings in the same division in the same university. That has been true all of our professional careers and has worked out pretty well for us. I had already known some of the faculty members here and one I did my residency with. I had met some of the more senior faculty members at meetings. One of the faculty members who is involved with the program into which my wife was hired really liked her, and when the positions came open, they called us.
>
> My fellowship director knew I was looking, and he is a friend of the chairman here, and the chairman called me up.
>
> I found the job through the doctor I trained with in my fellowship. My old boss and new boss had been friends for twenty years.

The successful candidate in a senior search explained his side of the effort in this way:

> In short, I had been at [previous school] for a long time, and I did not think things were moving the way I wanted them to move, so I made it clear to some people that I was looking outside. So the word got around that I was available. In the meantime, the person who was chief here left, and they had this position. They [the department] appointed an outside committee to evaluate the position, and I happened to know the people on the committee, and their recommendation was to approach me. So they called me to see if I was interested, and I was.

There was no discernible difference between the search to fill a tenure-track position and the search to fill a position that was not tenure-eligible. The same methods were used and the same sources were tapped. Neither did the search process differ in the case of basic scientists. These Ph.D. assistant professors made comments that were similar to the M.D.s quoted above:

> In a sense I may have created the position for myself. I met the person who recruited me at a meeting, and he heard a lecture I gave. He contacted me the first time before I took the job in industry, and then we had a chance meeting later and he offered me another job. And it seemed more attractive then.
>
> I was doing a gastroenterology postdoc here because my wife was here—she's an engineer at [a local industry]. I was doing some flow cytometry, and the person who was training me in hematology oncology told me of this position that he had become aware of through his contact with the surgeons. They were looking for someone who knew immunology and flow cytometry.
>
> Well, I have a joint appointment in internal medicine and cell biology, and I initiated the job myself. I created a space for myself by approaching the necessary people to continue my research with rheumatology and continue teaching in anatomy.

EVALUATING THE CANDIDATES

It was not clear whether search procedures limited applicant pools or expected applicant pools dictated search procedures, but even where a more traditional search was conducted, the result was a small applicant pool for a faculty position—fewer than ten candidates in most instances. This was in stark contrast to the arts and sciences scene, where the normal number of applicants for a position ranged from 50 to 200.

The short-listed junior candidates from these traditional search pools, as well as most of the specifically recruited individuals, were subsequently involved in a process closely resembling that found in the arts and sciences, but with another sharp difference: Letters of recommendation—a critical factor in an arts and sciences search—were a formality in the medical search, often obtained after an offer in order to satisfy institutional requirements for the candidate's dossier. New appointees proved to be the best source of information about this feature of the recruiting process, and these were typical comments (from different specialties and schools): "Afterwards I got letters for them"; "They asked for letters afterward for the dossier"; "After the offer we got all the formal stuff, paperwork"; "After I got the job I arranged for three letters of recommendation."

All of the candidates reported providing a c.v.—the basic starting point for evaluation in the arts and sciences as well—and the search usually began with an invitation to visit the department. The inclusion of the specifically recruited individuals reveals the dual purpose of the evaluation process: gaining the department's approval of a new colleague and selling the job. A chairman described the visit of a prospective assistant professor in these words:

> He wanted to work with me, and he came to visit to get to know the others for a better understanding of the training program. It was my decision, but there were two other faculty members in the section that I wanted him to meet. I knew the people he had trained with, and we just had him come here to make sure he was compatible.

Procedural elements of the visit varied widely, but in all cases, the candidate interviewed with members of the department. In a substantial number of cases (more than half), the candidate interviewed with members of other departments as well, in those areas in which the new faculty member would be interacting professionally.

The "job talk," a standard fixture of an arts and sciences search, was replaced by giving seminars or participating in rounds, but in only about a third of the hiring situations. The attitude of the majority was expressed by a chairman of surgery in this way:

> I don't ask them to give a talk because it's my job to determine an individual's capabilities, qualifications, capacities, etc. That obviously requires interviewing of the individual and feedback from others who have interviewed, and requires me to call and snoop around to get information about the individual, but I feel that it's unfair to impose on that person to have to talk—it's a "show me" attitude. I am recruiting somebody; I don't want to make them uncomfortable.

Another standard item of the arts and sciences search, however, was replicated in the medical search—engaging in assorted forms of social interaction that encouraged additional scrutiny by both parties. As one chairman told me, "Lunch is having the candidate checked out by a valued colleague, someone I can trust."

The prospective junior candidate rarely met the dean (in only 10 percent of the cases), and my question about meeting the dean drew the response from one chairman that "assistant professors don't meet deans." He continued:

> Associate and full get to meet deans because we need support from the dean's office. We need them to know that the department is moving, and we want the senior person interviewing to know that he's important to us.

Almost all of the new junior faculty members described an evaluation process that was "very informal," and of course many added, "They knew me." Perhaps the ultimate informality was expressed by an assistant professor of medicine in the southwest: "The division chief and his wife, two other division members with their spouses, and my wife and I met at a taco place and drank some beer."

For another assistant professor, switching from a hospital appointment, the process was anticlimactic:

> The chief just said to me that, we have this job; I said, "Does that mean I'm being offered a job;" he said, "Well, yes." It was a big change in my life, and you would expect to get a big letter and so forth. By the time I got back to him, he had already put it in the works with the administrator.

Presumably reflecting knowledge of the department gained after the fact, another assistant professor ascribed the informality to disinterest:

> I was interviewed by the chief and the chairman and that was pretty much it. This is a funny department. Everybody minds their own business—there are little fiefdoms and little sections, so one hand doesn't know or care what the other hand is doing.

More structure was present in a few recruiting visits; this account from an assistant professor of pediatrics was typical of those situations:

> I came on the night before, and they picked me up at the airport and took me to the hotel and then picked me up for dinner and picked me up the next morning. I went on rounds with one physician and had lunch with all of the physicians in the section. I had interviews with several people in pediatrics, medicine, and pathology. On the second visit, I met with the dean and the head of the coagulation lab.

Selling the job was especially important in the senior recruitment. Departments engaged in "courting" senior candidates—as a professor of medicine said, "In some ways it really is like a courtship." In a prestigious department of pediatrics, the chairman told me this:

> We were selling the opportunity. He was a pediatrician working in a research environment, and he wanted to come back to an environment that had a clinical arena. We offered him the view of what was available in a clinical institution with very heavy commitment to academic medicine and the freedom to continue with his own research in an environment where he could interact collegially with committed and bright people. He knew what was available, knew the national scene. Basically what we offer in this pediatrics department is a very large clinical base in a preeminent hospital that is successful on a fiscal level and can support the program. He could have the best of both worlds here—university identity and clinical identity, with strong support for the pediatrics program from the hospital.

Most senior candidates made multiple visits (this was true for many of the junior candidates as well), and another chairman of pediatrics talked about the final stages of discussion about the job:

> At this point the visit becomes very hand tailored, to the specific academic background and relations possible across the medical center in the broadest sense—research collaborative efforts that she might wish to be involved in, new programs to be initiated that we could begin exploring, various contacts. I spent a very lengthy period of time with her working through lunch in this office.

The search for a new chair might take a different turn, especially in a troubled department, as in this case recounted by a professor of anesthesiology:

> We all knew the candidates well. They wanted specifics about problems in the department that they had heard about, from members of the department and from our recent review—they were given a full copy of the document. They had a good idea of the problems. The other thing was that they had to be made aware of the opportunities.

And finally, there was the courtship involving the spouse employment issue (of which there were several instances in the sample). The recruitment of a professor of radiology took place in this way:

> It was a matter of selling him on the job. We made a package deal for the family—his wife is also in the department. We brought them in, showed them the campus. We showed them the town, etc. We had him talk with people in orthopedics and rheumatology and many people in radiology. And the dean talked to him—and if the dean knows we're really interested in somebody good, he does a selling job for us too.

On the senior candidate's part, the process was viewed as hard work. This search for a chair was described by the successful participant as a very thorough operation:

> The first day they picked me up at 6:10 A.M. and dropped me back at the hotel at 10:10 that night. The tail end of the first day was dinner, but it was with the search committee. I made two major visits where I was being looked at along with other people. The only parts of those that involved "selling" were discussions with the dean and the chairman of medicine. Out of those four days of interviews, the rest were unquestionably a drilling of me as to approaches. There were different roles of course: The search committee had to find the best candidate, but it was the dean's job to make sure that the best candidate took the job. It was really part of a viable competition. It was very clear that it was not a recruitment effort; if anything, it was going to boot camp. I've looked at several chairmanships before, and this was clearly the most grueling process.

Along the same lines, a professor described his three visits and then added, "It was like a beauty contest—you get a score for it."

Other senior people illustrated recruiting situations where the candidate appeared to have more control:

> There were various interviews, requested by *me*, with members of the department.

> I came and visited, and then I said, thanks, but I think I'll stay in Baltimore. The chairman called me and said, "Don't say no; tell us what it would take to bring you here."
>
> It evolved. They didn't know what I wanted, and I wasn't sure what they would provide. The minimum that I required was not quite what they appreciated. I was not satisfied with a tenured professorship or even an endowed chair—that wasn't the issue. It was important that a well-supplied lab would be immediately mine and any deficiencies would be immediately dealt with in terms of resources. I insisted on a certain amount of hard research money that the institution would provide. I insisted on a number of appointments and adequate space. If I didn't have that I wouldn't be here.

The recruiting of a basic scientist was conducted in essentially the same manner as that of the clinical scientist, and the applicant pools were, in most cases, no larger. In one junior search in obstetrics and gynecology, there were about 100 applicants; in three others, numbers ranged from ten to twenty, and in four junior searches and one senior search there were more than one applicant but fewer than five. But, as in the M.D. appointments, the single-applicant situation predominated (in twenty-two Ph.D. appointments, or 70 percent of the total), with almost half of those (nine) having moved to the faculty immediately after the doctorate or from a postdoctoral or adjunct position in the institution.

Except for the absence of a mention of clinical work, the comments displayed the same patterns as had been found in the comments about M.D. recruitments. These were examples from chairmen of family medicine, pathology, and obstetrics and gynecology:

> We do multiple interviews—cancer center, statisticians in this department, associate dean. Traditionally, we don't ask them to give a talk.
>
> I met the candidates the night before for dinner, and the next day they had a gauntlet of interviews with full professors and some associate professors—six or seven. They presented a seminar for the department and other members of the school. After the seminar they came back and spent some time with me; I got down to the nitty-gritty of lab space and what kinds of commitments they would like to see from me.

> The screening was essentially done by the division chief and myself. On the visit he [the candidate] met with me, with the division chief, and with two others in the department, and with some people in the basic science departments. He gave a seminar that was open to the basic sciences people. He visited the lab, met with the dean, and we had the usual social stuff.

Again, as in the initial recruiting, the Ph.D. appointees referred to the evaluation process in much the same terms as had the M.D. faculty members:

> I visited and interviewed. It's like "The Color of Your Parachute"—tell them what they need, and they'll hire you.
>
> I dealt mainly with the chief and the chairman. The chairman said to me, "What do you want?" So I mentioned several things. He suggested that I put down on paper what I needed and what I wanted to do, and I did that, and things just happened.

CHANGES IN THE RECRUITING PROCESS

Experienced chairs were helpful in identifying changes that had occurred in recruiting over the years, both in procedures and participants. Specialization and consequent complexity was a recurring theme in their comments; the following examples are from a department of psychiatry in one of the top-ranked schools and a department of otolaryngology in a lower-ranked school:

> It was easier when I started because whatever there was of quality out there we needed it. After a certain point we filled certain roles so that there are some people out there now for whom we don't have slots. At this point we would love to have a child development researcher—have been looking for a couple of years and haven't found the right person yet. Our searches have become much more focused, managed more carefully.
>
> Training programs have become a lot more focused so you have to be careful about the match between what you want and what the candidate has. You have to make sure that they have tracked themselves in a way that fits your need.

Growth in certain fields has also affected the way that the chair views recruiting. For this chairman of obstetrics and gynecology the task has developed in size and nature:

> I was chairman when I had six faculty members, and the department was fully staffed. This department now has thirty to forty, with several openings; we are never fully staffed. There is also a great change in the field with growing enthusiasm for research.

For a chairman of psychiatry, the recruiting process had changed only slightly but with some improvement:

> When I first started recruiting twenty years ago, it was much more word of mouth. You could rapidly determine who were the best people across the country. What has hung on is the network. But it is more rigorous now, not as pedantic and silly as it was about five years ago.

The rise and fall of medical specialties has also affected recruiting, as noted here by chairmen of radiology and psychiatry:

> Radiology has become much more academic. Twenty years ago people went to radiology when they couldn't get into other specialties, but we are now recruiting the top candidates into this specialty. There is more science in the specialty.
>
> Psychiatry has changed drastically in twenty years. We get candidates with much better academic qualifications, but there is a lot of ambivalence about academic careers in psychiatry, particularly because of the lack of certainty about research funding.

Faculty candidates, too, have changed. There was a general agreement that "people are differently trained, for academic work," but there was disagreement as to the degree and manifestation of change, as reflected in these comments:

> The candidates today are better trained because now everyone is a subsubspecialist, but as far as totality, they are no better than in the past.

> I don't know about "better," but it is a much more specialized kind of person than I had previously. Particularly now we are getting M.D.s with cell and molecular biology training.

> The people are incredibly good today. It's a combination of better training and changes in the field and changes in the rest of the medical fields—the interventional fields are interesting and complex. The majority of us feel we wouldn't get into our own departments today.

> There is no change in the candidates—they are better but only in the sense that the amount of training that people are obtaining before getting faculty positions is increasing every decade, but the quality has been superb right along.

The changes perceived in the training of candidates were not lacking in downside; negative effects were seen along with the positive. A long-time chairman of medicine at a top-ranked school noted:

> Candidates are more specialized, trained in narrower and narrower areas. Also, they are less interested in general clinical internal medicine. Internal medicine is becoming like a collection of small Balkan states.

AFFIRMATIVE ACTION

Certainly a change in recruiting procedure has been effected through affirmative action statutes and regulations in the past twenty years. But, as was the case in the arts and sciences, department heads did not think that affirmative action has had any substantive effect. About 85 percent of the respondents considered affirmative action to be largely a matter of formalities, having little or no real effect on recruiting. In the words of a chairman of psychiatry at a top-ranked school:

> We fill out the forms, certainly periodically we advertise, contact appropriate institutions and training directors, but it hasn't otherwise affected the search. Our representation of women is good; we have several senior professors who are women. We've had our fair share of blacks, but there are very, very few in psychiatry. We have a fair share of Hispanics at the training level but not attendings. Affirmative action hasn't really affected the

process except that we are more likely to advertise—but the quality of applicants one gets from ads is typically terrible.

Lack of results were remarked on universally:

> We are an affirmative action institution, and we have a very active affirmative action program, and so we advertised widely—not very successfully. It is not the most effective or efficient way of recruiting.
>
> You have to go through the process, but there were no minorities or women applying. With the pool of applicants being what it was, there were no questionable calls to be made. No more women and minority candidates are actually produced.
>
> It's a pain in the butt. It's doubtful that it affects candidates at all. We pick on merit and don't think about sex or color.

Many chairmen considered it just part of the routine—the "Mickey Mouse" that one went through to get a position filled. These were typical comments:

> We advertise. Once you choose to hire somebody, you fill out forms.
>
> We meet the paperwork needs.
>
> Well, there are forms to be filled out.
>
> I haven't been involved since I'm not getting money from anyone. I suppose I'd have to jump through those hoops if I were. I think it's all window dressing.

On the other hand, there were a few chairmen who thought that affirmative action was useful, albeit not effective, in the recruiting process:

> The letters that the committee sent out for nominations, for example, asked us to name women and minority candidates. I gave them names of two women, and it made me think about it, so I think it was effective, although neither of the women was as strong as [the successful candidate].

> Affirmative action advertising has no effect on the applicant pool, but I am in favor of process, and there is no doubt in my mind that some searches are totally against the guidelines and need to be stopped. But I honestly think that it is a bureaucratic requirement that doesn't change who the appointee happens to be.
>
> It makes it infinitely more time-consuming, but over the years has led to a more careful search. As far as candidates are concerned, it probably does not make any difference.

A chairman of radiology pointed out that a department's commitment was the more important factor in recruiting women and minorities:

> Well, affirmative action laws and regulations have changed the process to some extent, but it's still the old boy and girl network. Affirmative action works because we would like to have more blacks and more women, but it's not because somebody forces it. When somebody forces you, you try to find elegant ways to resist.

In sum, this chapter has identified a number of conditions affecting medical faculty recruitment: extensive use of an internal market and the presence in the market of women, minorities, and basic scientists, as well as the uncertainty of research funding and internal demographics. Decisions to recruit are frequently made by a department head, who may also be heavily involved in the recruiting, thus reinforcing his or her influence on the department. The decision itself is often tied to new or expanded programs, some fueled by new technology or research, others by patient care needs. The search for faculty members is generally informal at the junior level, involving small numbers, and relying heavily on an internal labor market and external networks; at the senior level, the search is wide and carefully constructed, and is more likely to result from a replacement need. And the locus of professional identity remains in the faculty itself, such that medical school or university administrations and institutional programs such as affirmative action have little effect on the search process.

The essence of medical faculty recruitment, especially the element of uncertainty and the importance of the departmental environment, have been essentially summarized by a long-time chief of cardiology:

> Recruiting is an impossible job to do well. I never know who's good until they've been here for awhile. I usually recruit knowing

what I want and I know what we need, where we're strong—and I recruit through the universe in which I function. I know people all over the world and up the street, and I use all of those contacts. Recruiting here is always an offshoot of some talent that's missing in our program. But I never cease to be amazed at how poor talent scouting is as an art. Talent happens after you get the person in the environment.

Chapter 4

Making Choices in Academic Medicine

> I chose academic medicine because I'm a glutton for punishment! You get to do all types of things and when you get tired of one thing, there is something else to do. Teaching is wonderful—I enjoy the contact with residents and medical students. I think it is the best of all possible worlds.
>
> Assistant Professor of Neurology

Populating this best of all possible worlds has been accomplished by selection among alternatives at various times and by various people. First, there are the initial choices made by the medical faculty member to attend medical school and to concentrate on a specialty area. Then there is the choice to enter academic medicine, which is frequently accompanied by being chosen as a likely prospect in the course of medical education. Finally, there are the organizational choices, interacting with the individual, that result in specific placement in jobs and institutions. This chapter, therefore, explores the circumstances of choice that affect staffing in medical academia.

INITIAL CAREER CHOICES

An important factor for any consideration of intervention to influence the attraction of academic medicine is the timing of the initial career decisions. The 143 new M.D. faculty members who were interviewed in this study furnished a rather surprising pattern in choosing to attend medical school, an expected one for the specialty decision, and mixed results on academic medicine (Table 4.1).

The surprise came from the large proportion (more than half) of the respondents who said that they had really known before they went to college—many in fact before high school—that they wanted to be doctors. An intuitively reasonable premise for this inclination would be the existence of parents or other close relatives in medicine, but this proved inadequate: 20 percent of the seventy-four faculty members who decided on medical school before college and 15 percent of the sixty-nine who did not had one or more parents or older siblings in medicine. (The difference between the percentages is not statistically significant at the .05 level.) Rather, the reasons given for the early choice were highly individual, but reflected a general fascination with science. From the experiment gone awry to the influence of the media, these comments from an associate professor and three assistant professors illustrated an early interest in science:

Table 4.1
Timing of Career Choices

Decision/ Time	Specialty Group									
	Medical		Surgical		Behavioral		Hospital-based		Total	
	No.	%	No.	%	No.	%	No.	%	No.	%
To attend Medical School										
Before college	31	51.7	22	55.0	2	22.2	19	55.9	74	51.7
During college	23	38.3	16	40.0	5	55.6	12	35.3	56	39.2
Other	6	10.0	2	5.0	2	22.2	3	8.8	13	9.1
Total	60	100.0	40	100.0	9	100.0	34	100.0	143	100.0
To select specialty										
Before medical school	13	21.7	6	15.0	2	22.2	2	5.9	23	16.1
During medical school	42	70.0	33	82.5	7	77.8	23	67.6	105	73.4
Other	5	8.3	1	2.5			9	26.5	15	10.5
Total	60	100.0	40	100.0	9	100.0	34	100.0	143	100.0
To enter academic medicine										
Before medical school	7	11.7	1	2.5					8	5.6
During medical school	17	28.3	12	30.0	1	11.1	4	11.8	34	23.8
During residency	18	30.0	26	65.0	4	44.4	17	50.0	65	45.5
During fellowship	6	10.0			1	11.1	4	11.8	11	7.7
Other	12	20.0	1	2.5	3	33.3	9	26.5	25	17.5
Total	60	100.0	40	100.0	9	100.0	34	100.0	143	100.0

Note: Percent totals adjusted for rounding.

In the sixth grade, I did an experiment in nutrition using mice, water, and mouse food. I gave one mouse water and the other mouse food, and the mouse that I gave water to died. I dissected it and discovered that its intestines were all glued together. What had happened was that I had built it a pretty little house with pink paper and had glued it all together, and the mouse had been so hungry it ate the paper and glue and that was what killed it. So my experiment failed because the water and the mouse food had nothing to do with it.

I decided on medical school in grade school; I'm not sure why. I loved science, and we did a project on the human body in my fourth grade science class that I liked very much.

I decided on medical school in the seventh grade. I did a series of reports on the body. I was fascinated by the human skeleton. (Initially, I wanted to go into nursing, but a counselor in high school steered me toward medical school.)

I decided probably in the eighth or ninth grade. My interest in research on humans was really sparked at that time—exposure in the press at that time was high profile—aeronautics, great advances in medicine, such as heart transplants.

Practical experience in the health care field at an early age played a role for several faculty members. These three assistant professors reported that influence:

I decided in the sixth grade, I think. Many of my parents' friends were physicians, and a close friend of the family one day just said, why don't you try it? So I started scrubbing in surgery with a friend and continued all through junior high school. Back then (1959–1960), litigation wasn't an issue and the nursing staff was always happy to have an extra body come in and help.

I went to Hunter College High School, which was an all-girls' school, very career oriented. We could graduate at the end of the eleventh grade or stay another year and do academics. So I did that, and I was able to do research at Lenox Hill Hospital that last year of high school.

I was one of those driven sorts of people who were probably pretty boring in high school. My pediatrician and a surgeon who fixed my broken foot were inspiring to me. I began to volunteer at a general hospital and worked there all through high school.

Among women, there was a certain amount of resistance to traditional choices displayed, as well as a decision for medicine made early in life. These were comments from three women assistant professors:

> When I was in high school, there were a group of six of us, and we all decided we would take different parts of the body and open up shop! Mom said, oh, you're going to be a nurse—I said, no, medical school. The woman thing was not a consideration.
>
> I decided on medical school when I was a child. I think if anything, it was the resistance that I felt twenty-five years ago when people would say, oh, don't you want to be a nurse, and it just made me that much more determined that I was going to show them.
>
> I decided on medical school about eighth grade. I come from a very religious family, Methodist, the oldest of seven, and I had read this book about a practicing missionary, and I told my mom, that's what I'm going to be—a doctor. The dean of girls at my high school tried to talk me out of it, but I was insistent.

Articulation of the desire to be a doctor was not so clear-cut for all respondents. Many had been determined about their objective to enter medicine from a young age but could not connect their determination to specific thoughts or incidents. These three assistant professors felt guided primarily by instinct:

> I remember being five and wanting to go to medical school—my mother has my kindergarten report card that proves it. I don't know why. I remember that my parents gave me a nurse's kit for Christmas one year, and I threw a fit and insisted on a doctor's kit. I used to do surgery on my doll.
>
> I've always wanted to be a doctor. I have no idea why. It was just one foot in front of the other, day by day, and I ended up a doctor.
>
> I knew that I wanted to go to medical school since I was in high school. I don't know why. I can't tell, except that I had this

> attraction. I'd rather work on my gut feeling because I can't cheat on that.

And there was just a touch of levity in this assistant professor's response:

> I decided I wanted to be a doctor in the third grade. I had to start wearing glasses then, and everyone told me I could not be a pilot (honest!). But as I got older, I was attracted by the job independence, the financial security, the love of science, the chance to actually contribute to the fate of individual people on a personal basis. It was an outlet for a driven person who loves constant challenges.

As might be expected, in view of the fact that medical students must select a specialty in order to begin graduate medical education, the bulk of the respondent group said that they had selected the specialty in which they were now practicing during medical school—most in their last year. The small proportion who gave an "other" answer had switched specialties during training or after initial training; responses in this category offered insights into perceived differences between specialties, as in these remarks:

> I did medicine and surgery before I shifted to pathology. When I was a resident I felt that as a doctor you were always depending on a third person to tell you what the patient has. You run to the lab all the time to get the biopsy report. It occurred to me that the pathologist knew more than we did.
>
> In terms of research issues, obstetrics and gynecology is where medicine was ten years ago—and it is applicable to my own body, quite stimulating. My temperament is not as geared to internal medicine—rounding, discussing cases, *ad infinitum.* With the patient population in ob-gyn I could do something more concrete. I discovered that I really enjoy operating, working with my hands, developing finesse with techniques.
>
> I switched from internal medicine because of a combination of two factors: I felt that the intervention done by pediatricians can really have a more profound effect (because the kids are young), and I knew I was going to do academic medicine.

The other small group of respondents, who had decided on a specialty before they got to medical school, were influenced by childhood experiences. Having made an early decision on a specialty, they gave answers to the question of choice that frequently referred to subspecialty, as in these:

> As a child I always wanted to be a doctor. I had noticed the increased risk of heart disease in my family; when I was in high school I had seen a favorite aunt in cardiac arrest. I vowed to become a doctor and cure that disease. There were really no alternatives in my mind—it was always cardiology, and it was rhythm disorders that attracted me most.
>
> As far as medical school is concerned, in my family—well, growing up there was only one acceptable occupation! I rebelled for a brief period but got over that. I selected surgery my sophomore year of college. I just decided I wanted to be a brain surgeon. I had worked in the hospital with my father [an ophthalmologist] and liked the neuro system.
>
> I became a pediatrician because my grandfather was a pediatrician. But I wasn't quite sure what I wanted to do within pediatrics. Originally, I was interested in host defense, and I thought I would end up a cancer specialist or in infectious diseases. I took a course at NIH in rheumatology, and I discovered that those patients had all the things I was interested in without the stress of cancer or the parts of infectious disease that I don't care about.

Of the majority group who chose their specialty during medical school, the reasons for doing so were clustered in general categories of the influence of a mentor, a positive comparison with another specialty, and the intrinsic values of the specialty. Mentors were mentioned by many respondents; these comments were typical: "The faculty member I was closest to was a psychiatrist," "very positive influence of a neurologist with whom I did an elective," "a preceptor in surgery who impressed me." Two particularly compelling accounts from senior faculty members were these:

> Both medical school and pediatrics came out of a conversation with [a scientist] at Fermilab about physics and kids—that they were more fun than physics. I suppose it was because of him that my thinking was triggered along a totally different pathway.

> I decided on anesthesia my second year of medical school. I didn't even know what it was before I went to medical school. I had a series of lectures in pharmacology, and the man who gave the lectures on the pharmacology of anesthetics was extremely dynamic and simply made a superb presentation. Three of us who were in that class are now chairmen of anesthesia.

A comparative method led to decisions in several instances, sometimes in a negative sense, that is, eliminating what was not liked. Choices between radiology and ophthalmology, family and internal medicine (after dismissing surgical specialties), and medicine and ob-gyn were reported by these three assistant professors:

> I decided on radiology my last year of medical school. I was set on ophthalmology until about three months before leaving. I decided that I didn't want to work with patients that much, doing eye exams with people who wouldn't understand what was going on and so forth.
>
> I decided on medicine in medical school after my junior year. A lot of it had to do with what I didn't like. I hated ob-gyn and surgery. Originally I was going to do family practice, but I thought I would get a better education in general medicine.
>
> I was disappointed by internal medicine's pursuit of diagnosis and treatment as sociologic benefit. No matter how interesting a given problem was, if it was untreatable in a senile patient, I felt my effort was wasted. In ob-gyn I feel my work has significant socioeconomic impact.

The comparative method was extended by a small minority of the respondents to what might amount to flipping a coin. Here is an explanation of that process:

> My best friend and I lived in a nursing dorm, and we used to get a six-pack of beer and sit around in the evenings talking about what we were going to do and saying, "Do you really want to be a primary care physician?" (My father is a general practitioner.) After numerous discussions about it, we each decided to do a rotation in anesthesia and radiology. She went into radiology, and I did anesthesia. It was purely a logical decision. It just turned out that I happened to like it.

Another large group of respondents spoke about the special attractions of their fields. These are examples from radiology, obstetrics and gynecology, internal medicine, and surgery:

> There are two reasons that people go into radiology. It's become very exciting, one of the fastest growing specialties, advancing technology, a very exciting field. And a lot of people find they are not cut out to be in the clinical trenches. I was a good intern, but I couldn't stand working on the ward, handling the day-to-day responsibilities; I could never get it off my mind, people depending on you whether you were there or not. In radiology, when your day ends, your day ends.
>
> I liked endocrinology a whole lot as a medical student, and it was the ability to be in a specialty that would be involved with endocrinology and counseling as well as surgery and medicine. It is an interesting specialty, lots of ethical issues.
>
> Internal medicine is the area that has the most science in it—pathophysiology, the most cutting-edge research. I am more interested in why diseases occur and why treatment works.
>
> I interviewed both medical and surgical internships, but surgery was my final choice. I enjoy the opportunity to do something technical with my hands, felt that as a surgeon I could do anything an internist could do and have the advantage of doing something interventional. Plus you can almost always really help the patient. There are only a few areas in medicine where you can really cure or help substantially. I enjoy seeing patients, doing something for them and seeing the results.

After choice of specialty, the next (not necessarily the last) fork in the career path for the physician is the choice between academic medicine and other options—private practice, health maintenance organization, staff physician in varied settings, and so on. Although there was some movement between the university and the nonacademic setting in the sample, most of the respondents in the study had taken the academic road for reasons that showed a clear separation from other possibilities, perhaps owing at least partially to personality differences. An obstetrician suggested that "people who want to go into private practice are oriented that way before they get into medical school," and while the actual choice of academic medicine may not be so definitive as he implied, there does appear to be an orientation reflected in the respondents' primary reasons for choosing a university practice (Table 4.2).

Teaching and research were given as motivation for the choice in two-thirds of the cases (teaching was frequently a second choice for those first citing research, and research second for those giving teaching first). Occupying a distant third place was task variety, followed by the perceived higher quality of patient care in a university-affiliated hospital and the role of mentorship. "Other" responses were generally pragmatic in nature—"I wanted to get married to a medical student, and I needed a job" or, from a woman, "I wanted to integrate family life and career." A few respondents mentioned that their particular subspecialty required an academic setting, either because of its investigative nature or the need for the kind of referral base available in an academic medical center—examples were pediatric electrophysiology, pediatric hematology-oncology, and trauma surgery. (An interesting footnote on the similarity of medical academicians regardless of tenure status is the fact that a third of the group choosing research as the primary motivating factor were faculty members not on the tenure track.)

Table 4.2
Reasons for Choosing Academic Medicine

	Specialty Group									
Reason Given by Faculty Member	Medical		Surgical		Behavioral		Hospital-based		Total	
	No.	%	No.	%	No.	%	No.	%	No.	%
Teaching; continued learning, keeping up with new technologies and practices	16	26.7	17	42.5	4	44.4	14	41.2	51	35.7
Research, making scientific contributions	20	33.3	11	27.5	4	44.4	9	26.5	44	30.8
Variety in work; problems, challenges	14	23,3	5	12.5	1	11.1	4	11.8	24	16.8
Quality of clinical program	5	8.3	2	5.0			2	5.9	9	6.3
Faculty example, socialization	3	5.0	3	7.5			2	5.9	8	5.6
Other	2	3.3	2	5.0			3	8.8	7	4.9
Total	60	100.0	40	100.0	9	100.0	34	100.0	143	100.0

Note: Percent totals adjusted for rounding

Teaching is clearly the bug that bites a great many medical students and residents, turning them toward academic medicine, as these comments indicate:

> I think the main thing really is the ability to have an impact on people who are training. I enjoy seeing young people come through and developing them, helping them along. Instead of just practicing the state of the art, there's the idea that I might advance it.
>
> I like to teach. Here I have a fellow, such a well-trained guy, you can really leave a mark on him. Some day I would like to have my own department and train my own people. I admired the people who were in academics—they were not only good doctors but took the time to train me, shared their knowledge.
>
> At first I wasn't at all academic, and now I have become a hard core academic. I enjoy teaching, the different ideas we can use, contributing to science. It's a privilege to work as a physician, not a right; we have an obligation to contribute to the science we're using.

As for the affinity for research, especially clinical research, an M.D.-Ph.D. professor of pediatrics elaborated on his choice in this way:

> My own career has been somewhat transitional as a scientist who has passed through medicine—I don't see myself as a doctor who is doing scientific research, I see myself as a scientist who has passed through medicine. In the problems that we, as scientists interested in biological processes, deal with, we would like to focus on human disease, and the training as a physician is the most exhaustive and complete way of really learning about human biology. It's sort of pleasing to know how to help people, and I am happy in clinical work as a doctor. Man is the best study animal, we have the best genetics in man, we know the most about man—and that is medical school information.

Another professor of pediatrics also described the lure of scientific investigation centered on the patient:

> I went to Hopkins planning on going into private practice, working with handicapped children. One of the children I admitted had a rare metabolic disorder that was usually fatal, and I worked

out a treatment. I worked in the lab on that and then became more and more ensconced in academia.

Variety in day-to-day responsibilities was mentioned by several respondents as an attractive feature of academic medicine; the desire for variety seemed to accompany a strong feeling that the only way to stay well informed in the field was to be associated with an academic medical center. Of course, this feeling was often engendered during training—one assistant professor remarked that one year three out of four residents went into private practice, and the chairman threatened to close his residency program. But perhaps an "average" response explaining the attraction of academic medicine came from this assistant professor of obstetrics and gynecology:

> Well, I'm not exactly a dynamo in research so I really can't claim that I have a strong urge to be actively involved in a research setting. Money clearly isn't an issue. The best I can say is that the stimulation of having a constantly varying lifestyle professionally and the ability to be involved in real specific things, is that they outdraw other options. There is always the feeling that you will have big projects that will change the course of the profession. And there is a lot more of that going on than I would have thought.

ORGANIZATIONAL SELECTION

Given a group of persons who have identified themselves as interested in academic medicine, the clinical science department culls from its sources in a manner that continues the tradition of efficiency but with the introduction of a greater degree of democracy than existed in the earlier stages of recruitment. The chair acting alone in an appointment is a rarity, although the clinical chair can in no way be described as the "first among equals" common in arts and sciences thinking—his or her veto power is absolute but not exercised because this congress would never send a candidate forward who might be vetoed. In other words, the chair (or in some cases, the division chief, or a combination of the two) is sufficiently in control of the process to prevent either unpleasant surprises or palace uprisings.

Faculty members were involved to some degree in the selection decision in about 40 percent of the hiring departments. Several chairs expressed a sensitivity to their faculties in the actual selection of new faculty members that was not present in responses concerned with the earlier stages of recruiting, as reflected in these comments:

> Most interviewers write notes, but in any case I would speak to everybody [about the candidate]. I'm interested in getting as much concurrence as possible among the existing faculty.
>
> This is a small department. It is supposed to be a decision of the tenured faculty, but, in fact, we have the whole department get together. This was not a contentious appointment; there was general agreement.
>
> What I like to do is sort of not do things on my own for several reasons—one, I get less opposition, and I get reinforcement whether I'm right or not. It's like going into a harbor among buoys.
>
> It was a collaborative hiring decision—phone calls, discussion—rather informal.
>
> Well, the department is sort of a big happy family. We do these things by consensus in many cases.

Still, the oligarchical or dictatorial stance was well represented; a sampling follows:

> The hiring decision is really made by the executive committee in the department, which consists of the four most senior division chiefs. I won't go after a person until there is unanimity within this group.
>
> I told the executive committee I wanted to recruit him, and they gave me approval.
>
> Some members of the faculty write me letters, others come in and say the candidate was great or they weren't impressed. But it is the personal interaction that I have with the recruit that is the single most important factor as to whether I offer a job or not.
>
> I said to John [the division chief], who do you think is the best person, and she was the standout. We always get feedback from the people who interviewed—they fill out little sheets. But it's not a democracy!
>
> I made the hiring decision.

An exception to the selection decision made within the medical school department was the appointment based in an affiliated hospital. There, the major participants in the decision were likely to be the members of the hospital organization that paid the salary, or a large part of the salary, of the new faculty member. At the five Veterans Affairs hospitals in the sample, for example, appointments were made by the chief of service at the hospital "with the approval of the department chairman," after a search in which the medical school played a part. At hospitals other than V.A. hospitals, the relationships seemed more tenuous. Chairs commented: "I saw his vita but they selected him"; "the division of neurology at the hospital is fiscally independent, and the chief is independent as well"; the relationship with the hospital is "fairly distant." My impression from these and other comments was that paperwork was reviewed, and interviews may have taken place, but the selection decision took place outside the university—and that this was the case regardless of whether the appointment was or was not tenure-eligible.

Indeed, as in recruitment, there were no discernible differences in the selection process as between tenure track and nontenure track appointments, although the question of tenure track appears in this study as an area of institutional variance. In two of the schools (both top-ranked), almost all of the appointments were made to the tenure track; in two (one top-ranked), almost all of the appointments were not tenure-eligible; in the remaining two schools, the appointments were mixed (see Appendix B). The real status of these appointments, however, belies the apparent difference. In both of the top-ranked schools where tenure-track appointments were predominant, considerable movement off the track was reported (although university regulations in one case would seem to preclude such movement). A chairman of obstetrics and gynecology at one of the schools told me, "What happens is that they switch to the other track later, at the third or probably the sixth year point," and an associate dean at the other said, "We try to make a place for everybody." This stretching of the rules has been described as the result of tension created by the influence on university regulations of faculty senates; such bodies, dominated by arts and sciences faculty members, were believed by medical academicians to have little understanding of or tolerance for the demands of applied science in a medical school.

Whatever the cause, the effect was a blurring of boundaries between faculty classifications that was reflected in a lack of difference in the recruiting process. At one of the top-ranked schools, a chairman of radiology succinctly stated an opinion common in the clinical sciences:

> We make very little distinction between tenured and untenured faculty. Most people in the department don't know whether they have tenure or not. Nobody, when you come down to it, has tenure.

The actual authority to appoint at the assistant professor level was held by the department chair in four of the six schools; at the other two, junior appointments were referred to one or more review committees above the departmental level. All senior appointments were subjected to review beyond the department, and the authority in many of these appointments rested with a dean, or even a provost, depending on the impact of the appointment on the medical school or the university as a whole. (Of course, the ultimate authority for faculty appointments was held at all of the schools by a governing board, but the board's action was a formality that implemented decisions made at other levels in the organization.)

BASES OF CHOICE: TWO PERSPECTIVES

The recruitment process is basically one of ensuring a good fit between the candidate and the department. But what are the ingredients of "fit"? There is, as one chairman of medicine admitted, "a lot of intuition." But department chairs talking about junior recruitments referred to research record, clinical ability (based on their own experience or that of colleagues they trusted), enthusiasm, experience in basic science (for M.D.s)—and especially, observed qualities, in the case of their former residents and fellows. This actual observation of candidates at work was a great advantage for the department contemplating faculty appointments and resulted in the judgments noted in these comments:

> We were impressed with his research ability and his training. He had presented papers at national meetings, had publications, had experience with MRI.
>
> She was unbelievably enthusiastic, bright-eyed, and energetic. I thought she would carry that kind of enthusiasm into clinical practice and sweep up other people in enthusiastic reaction to various projects.
>
> She was very good at the bedside and was doing very good research.

> She was interested in breast disease and had experience in molecular biology. She really filled the bill.
>
> His academic record. A combination of a first-rate neurology training program plus an absolutely first-rate neuro-ophthalmology program. Qualities that I—and all of the other department members—had observed when he was here as a resident.

In fact, early identification of faculty candidates during the residency has become increasingly important with accelerating subspecialization. The candidate's fit can be structured. As one chairman of obstetrics and gynecology said:

> More and more in these highly specialized areas we have to identify someone, help them to get training, because there are so few candidates for these subspecialties.

In the case of senior candidates, maturity and professional reputation were the important factors, along with financial and political skills. The strong influence of the external environment on the medical school is evidenced by these rationales for the appointment of senior faculty members:

> We needed somebody who could make the clinic go. This is becoming a much more difficult thing to do with the third party reimbursement problem.
>
> Trauma is unique. He knew this area very well with respect to trauma programs, multiple interface problems, city politics, paramedical units.
>
> She had national stature, had done work on national committees—a strong leader.
>
> He had independent NIH funding of a significant amount.

But perhaps the more telling definition of fit in this seller's market was obtained from the sought-after faculty members themselves. The 115 M.D. junior faculty members who were interviewed responded to the question of why they took that particular job in a variety of ways (Table 4.3).

Generally, the most frequently cited primary reason was geographic location, including desired proximity to family, location in the place

Table 4.3
Reasons for Taking Specific Junior Faculty Position

Reason Given by Junior Faculty Member	Specialty Group: Medical No.	%	Surgical No.	%	Behavioral No.	%	Hospital-based No.	%	Total No.	%
Geographic location (including spouse accommodations)	10	22.7	4	11.1	1	12.5	6	22.2	21	18.3
Individual research interests, protected time	6	13.6	8	22.2	2	25.0	1	3.7	17	14.8
Prestige in specialty of department, chair, or chief	1	2.3	7	19.4	2	25.0	7	25.9	17	14.8
Respect/liking for colleagues in department or section	5	11.4	2	5.6	1	12.5	7	25.9	15	13.0
Respect/liking for individual who recruited	6	13.6	6	16.7			2	7.4	14	12.2
Quality of clinical program, good place to practice	5	11.4	4	11.1	1	12.5	1	3.7	11	9.6
Specific program and/or challenge in department	6	13.6	1	2.8			1	3.7	8	7.0
Opportunities to specialize, teach	1	2.3	3	8.3	1	12.5	1	3.7	6	5.2
Balance or mix of research and clinical	3	6.8							3	2.6
Other	1	2.3	1	2.8			1	3.7	3	2.6
Total	44	100.0	36	100.0	8	100.0	27	100.0*	115	100.0*

*Total adjusted for rounding

where a spouse or significant other had or could get a job, or just a liking for the region. Respondents explained in these words:

> This job was close to my parents and brother. We wanted to be back in this area, although my husband came without a job.

> My husband wanted to stay in the area; he is an engineer. He had moved for my fellowship, and it was his turn. He's very happy in his job.

> My wife wanted to move to the East for family and school reasons. She is originally from the East. She was a nurse adminis-

trator, very good, but she went to chef school here, and she is now a chef.

I really don't want to live anywhere else.

The next two most popular reasons were related through the nature of academic prestige, which relies on research and published work. Fifteen percent of the respondents gave as their foremost reason for taking the job the compatibility of the department with their own research interests, combined with the willingness of the department to support their research through such actions as providing sufficient protected time (from clinical duties) to engage in research. Another 15 percent were attracted by the prestige in the specialty of the department as a whole or of senior individuals in the department, again related to their reputations as researchers. These were typical remarks:

> One of my goals is to develop a research program. This job gives me a lot of flexibility. I'm hired to do clinical medicine, and I'm not on a tenure track. They expect you to teach on the wards and give an occasional lecture, perhaps some faculty development work, and work with the internal medicine fellows. I only have five half days of clinical responsibility, and the remaining time I can use for research.
>
> The research potential was something—a definite 50 percent commitment to do research, protected time, and a lot of support from both the cardiac surgery section and the chairman of the department.
>
> The major appeal here for me is the commitment of this department to its junior faculty doing research and the quality of the medical center as a whole. There is an impressive research program here that has been developed by the chairman.
>
> Basically, I came because of the division chief and his reputation.
>
> It was the names. The chairman and his colleagues are very well known in our specialty.

At the next two levels of response frequency, individuals were also recognized, via the new faculty member's respect for colleagues or recruiters; many of these respondents were former residents or fellows who had stayed on in faculty positions. These were typical comments:

> First, I knew [the division chief] quite well, knew who I would be working for. (I wasn't directly in his lab but I was a nephrology fellow.) So that to me was very important.

> The real drawing card was [the division chief], extremely bright, energetic, personable, and somebody who it seemed to me would be good to have as a colleague.

Throughout the responses there was a thread of appreciation for the support or perceived support shown by the members of the hiring department, which was well expressed by this assistant professor:

> They gave me very good treatment when I came over to talk with them and have been very good to me since then. You can weather a lot of things if you feel someone wants you to succeed, and I feel that I have tremendous support here.

The senior faculty experience centered on opportunity and prestige. The twenty-eight M.D.s who were interviewed expressed as principal reasons for taking the job the challenge of building or developing the department or the prestige or quality of the department (Table 4.4).

Some of the new senior faculty members talked about rescuing troubled programs, as follows:

> If I was going back to academics, I wanted to go to a strong, well-known institution, but I'm also very programmatically and administratively oriented so I wanted a place that was in deep trouble administratively—I did not want to step into somebody else's shoes, I wanted to make my own shoes. This particular program was in trouble and this fit the bill perfectly.

> Because of the crisis in leadership, several people had left, and I had an opportunity to rebuild practically from scratch. The previous person had been very destructive for the unit and had left it demoralized. The resources are fair; they gave me everything I wanted.

Others referred to building on an already good program or using a welcoming environment, as in these remarks:

Table 4.4
Reasons for Taking Specific Senior Faculty Position

Reason Given by Senior Faculty Member	Specialty Group: Medical No.	%	Surgical No.	%	Behavioral No.	%	Hospital-based No.	%	Total No.	%
Opportunity to build, develop department or program in progressive environment	5	33.3	4	80.0			1	14.3	10	35.7
Academic quality, prestige of department or institution, research	7	46.7			1	100.0	2	28.6	10	35.7
Other	3	20.0	1	20.0			4	57.1	8	28.6
Total	15	100.0	5	100.0	1	100.0	7	100.0	28	100.0

> This place is very famous for pediatric rheumatology. I want a world-class pediatric rheumatology program, and they gave me the resources to build one.

> I would say I felt this was a better opportunity, number one, and number two, the people are more receptive to new ideas. Universities cannot live in the old traditional forms. This place is willing to move with the times. It is a more attractive environment.

The majority of the senior group was more homogeneous with respect to motivating themes, but the minority was more diverse, with almost a third of the respondents giving uniquely individualized responses. An example was the former voluntary faculty member, who said:

> I was in practice for a long time, a general internist. I started cutting back, and had a lot of time for refining tests, etc., that I had developed—and got the idea that the tests I was doing had something to do with hypertension. Now I see patients a half day a week on a limited consultation basis and spend the rest of my time in research. I thoroughly enjoyed my practice, but it was enough. I wanted to pursue some very exciting ideas that may make a difference some day.

There were two topics that recurred in the comments from both junior and senior faculty about choosing the job: the irrelevance of money to the decision and the relevance of the job's effect on family life. Several chairs had told me that spouse employment was a new and critical factor in recruiting, and this was borne out in the interviews with new appointees. In addition, a number of women had mentioned the compatibility of an academic job and family life. What was an unexpected feature, however, were the many comments made by men about job and family, as in these responses as to their reasons for taking the job given by two assistant professors and two associate professors:

> Primarily time at home. I don't want to spend my entire life in the hospital, and we are on call only about twice a month here.
>
> Convenience. The desire to spend more time with my two children.
>
> Mainly I came here for family reasons. We have two little children and wanted to be around one set of [our] parents.
>
> I had a one-year-old, and I wanted to spend more time at home.

That salary was a nonissue was specifically mentioned by many of the new faculty members: From an assistant professor of obstetrics and gynecology, "I took a $200,000 cut in pay"; from a professor of pediatrics, "I took a 20 percent cut in salary to come here"; from an assistant professor of medicine, "I took a 50 percent salary cut to come here"; from an associate professor of anesthesia, "I probably make between a half and two-thirds of what I would be making in private practice."

For those faculty members who had come from another job (as opposed to residency or fellowship), the "pull" factors to the new position were much stronger than any "push" factors from the old. But there were patterns in the push factors that did exist, and these could be identified from junior faculty responses: strife or reorganization in the old department; space and growth potential lacking; no or insufficient protected time; stagnation—having stayed on after residency or fellowship; or the private practice was too busy, and there was no time for research. Senior respondents echoed the themes at a different level; for example, the organizational difficulties were likely to be institutional or governmental rather than departmental, frustrations were largely intellectual, and personal motivators such as divorce were present.

THE PRESTIGE FACTOR

It is well known that doctoral prestige plays an important role in the selection of Ph.D.s for junior faculty positions in the arts and sciences. The prestige factor is present as well in junior appointments to the clinical science faculty (Table 4.5).

Slightly more than 60 percent of the new junior faculty members in the study earned their medical degrees at the top fifty medical schools—31 percent at the top nineteen. But a more adequate gauge of the prestige factor for the medical faculty is in the residency; 72 percent of the appointments went to those who had completed residencies at the top fifty schools, and almost half to doctors who had completed residencies at the top nineteen schools. Residency training is also apparent as a gateway to the faculty of the school in which training takes place; 32

Table 4.5
Origins of New Junior Faculty, by School Ranking*

School of Origin	In Schools Ranked in Top 19 (N=98)	In Schools Ranked 20 to 50 (N=44)	Total (N=142)**
Ranked 1 to 19:			
M.D.	35	9	44
Residency 1	58	9	67
Residency 2	11	1	12
Fellowship 1	42	10	52
Fellowship 2	4		4
Ranked 20 to 50:			
M.D.	26	16	42
Residency 1	13	22	35
Residency 2	4	3	7
Fellowship	19	12	31
Ranked below 50:			
M.D.	21	13	34
Residency 1	11	3	14
Residency 2	2	2	
Fellowship	5	2	7
Not Ranked:			
M.D.	16	6	22
Residency 1	12	4	16
Residency 2	4		4
Fellowship	11	3	14

* Cole and Lipton (1977). Schools not ranked are either schools not included in the Cole and Lipton rankings of 87 U.S. medical schools or foreign medical schools.

** Residency information was not available on 10 new appointments.

percent of the new appointees had completed first, second, or both residencies at the hiring institution.

The pattern of credential prestige is still present at the senior level, as shown in Table 4.6.

The M.D. had been earned at one of the top fifty medical schools by 65 percent of the newly appointed associate and full professors, and the residency had been completed at one of those fifty schools by 75 percent of the appointees. In addition, 65 percent of the new faculty members who had come from academic positions had been employed at top-fifty schools. In terms of perceived prestige, this last figure would be increased by a number of appointees who came from well-reputed research institutes or foreign schools.

Table 4.6
Origins of New Senior Faculty, by School Ranking*

School of Origin	In Schools Ranked in Top 19 (N=21)	In Schools Ranked 20 to 50 (N=13)	Total (N=34)
Ranked 1 to 19:			
M.D.	5	5	10
Residency 1	14	9	23
Residency 2		3	3
Fellowship	10	5	15
Faculty	11	7	18
Ranked 20 to 50:			
M.D.	8	4	12
Residency 1	2		2
Residency 2	2		2
Fellowship	1	2	3
Faculty	4		4
Ranked below 50:			
M.D.	6	3	9
Residency 1	2		2
Residency 2	1		1
Fellowship		1	1
Faculty		1	1
Not Ranked:			
M.D.	2	1	3
Residency 1	3	4	7
Residency 2	2	1	3
Fellowship	3	1	4
Faculty/Other	6	5	11

* Cole and Lipton (1977). Institutions not ranked are foreign medical schools or nonacademic institutions such as the National Institutes of Health; figures also include 3 appointments in the top-19 group and 2 in the 20-50 group made from private practice.

A finding reported in the literature that is not supported here is an observed tendency for faculty members to move within a like group of schools. None of the new senior faculty members appointed in the group ranked 20 to 50 came from that group, although four of those appointed in the top-15 group did, and seven former top-15 faculty members took jobs in the 20-to-50 group. (Of course, these are small numbers from which no firm conclusions can be drawn, but there is an anecdotal sense that today there is a greater flexibility in mobility for experienced faculty members than had existed in past years.)

Beyond the implications for prestige in the faculty selection decision, Tables 4.5 and 4.6 serve to illustrate another aspect of academic prestige—that deriving from the complexity of subspecialization in medical fields. Of the 176 total M.D. appointments, one-fifth of the new faculty members had completed more than one residency, and three-quarters had completed a fellowship.

CLOSING THE DEAL

The recruitment process in academic medicine is interactive between recruiting organization and recruited individual to the extent that it is difficult to establish a line where an "offer" is made. Nevertheless, the formality of offer and acceptance was required in all of the departments studied, again varying in execution by institution. As mentioned earlier, chairs were essentially authorized to offer and appoint at the assistant professor level at four of the schools. At another, chair and dean acted jointly, and at the sixth institution, all offers were reviewed by a medical school committee although the chair had the authority to write a conditional offer letter.

Again, the autonomy of the clinical department in appointments derived from financial autonomy, as indicated by a chairman of anesthesia who said, "The salary comes out of clinical earnings, and so I have considerable autonomy there." And chairs have various internal methods for handling finances, as was usefully illuminated by this respondent:

> I made the offer. I have a finance committee that I talk to—when I started in the department, our budget was $700,000 a year, and now it's $12 million. We struck a reasonable salary level and agreed to put him on some time early in order to cover moving expenses.

The department may also have a degree of independence with respect to the offer of a senior appointment, although in all cases in this study, it was necessary for academic credentials to be approved for formal appointment. This might cost the department some time in discussion after all other terms and conditions were agreed on, as in this instance:

> He wanted the professorial title, and we recommended him as a tenured professor, but the university committee split when they reviewed his credentials. Some felt that he was not someone who had international recognition, and some felt that he was. The committee would have approved appointment as associate professor with tenure, but we discussed it with him, and he wanted the professorial title; so we put him through as nontenure track.

The negotiation involved in offering and accepting was also woven into the larger recruiting process, culminating in the final stages in agreement on such matters as protected time, clinical work, space and equipment, startup funds, support staff. Typical was this explanation given by a chairman of surgery:

> I made the offer on her second visit. She's a tough kid. She set forth what she wanted. This is very important because it tells you what you're going to get, right? Items were 40 percent protected time, opportunities for patient care, lab space, startup funds. She did not make an initial salary request; I offered a salary, and she asked for more, and I gave it to her.

There were the usual academic situations of a senior person negotiating for people: "He was part of a senior woman's recruitment"; "He brought his team from UCLA with him (two people)"; "I made a commitment to hire two to three other people." At the junior level, moving expenses and housing assistance were worked out in various ways. In radiology, there was frequently negotiation of "time on the machines."

In the recruitment of an assistant professor (not tenure eligible) over a period of time, his chairman said:

> He interviewed when he was in training, and he needed financial support for his second fellowship. So I gave him a loan that he will be able to pay back during the next two years.

In another discussion of a specific junior recruitment, a chairman of pediatrics offered general thoughts on negotiation:

> It is my experience that these decisions are usually made on the basis of mutuality, not on the basis of money. We want the work here to be professionally exciting, and we give them support in their research, and if that doesn't interest them we don't want them. We gave her research support, a technician, space, equipment, protected time. We give our candidates anything that's realistic, or they won't be productive.

Notwithstanding the formal framework of offer and acceptance in place at the hiring institutions, new junior faculty members reported a somewhat less exacting procedure. Offers were made verbally during a visit or by phone shortly thereafter; follow-up letters sometimes arrived after the faculty member had started work, entailing some risk, as recognized by this assistant professor:

> They called me at the end of November, and I came in January. I accepted verbally before there was anything in writing, so I was here for almost four months before an offer was put in writing. I did not know what title I would carry. I guess I took sort of a calculated risk.

Informality was also the order of the day in many cases of a resident or fellow moving to a faculty position, as reported in these responses:

> There was nothing formal, no contract. They expect you to continue and show up the next day [after completing the residency].
>
> It was quite unofficial. The director of my laboratory basically told me that everything would be taken care of. There was nothing official until after July, when I "officially" started.

As in most other matters with respect to medical faculty recruiting, funding sources played a role in the offer mechanism as well, as in these situations in departments of medicine and surgery:

> [The offer was communicated] informally by an associate professor of cardiology and the head of magnetic resonance. They

> were supporting me until I had my own funds, which I now have from NIH and the Heart Association.
>
> It was completely verbal, followed shortly by a letter from the director of the hospital. I didn't get an appointment letter from the university for about a year.

Negotiation at the acceptance stage was reported by more than half of the junior faculty members—58.6 percent, almost equally apportioned between men (58.8 percent of the total of ninety-seven male appointees who were interviewed) and women (58.3 percent of the thirty-six women). Negotiated items were generally those mentioned by the chairs, with a special emphasis on protected time (which in some cases had been covered satisfactorily in theory but had not actually worked out very well in practice). Other items were a computer, maternity leave, elimination of an unwanted trauma rotation—and one enterprising assistant professor of obstetrics and gynecology successfully negotiated a phone in his car.

Several of those who had not negotiated their employment adequately expressed regrets. In a tiny office shared with two other people, an assistant professor of pediatrics ruefully remarked that she had failed to ask for a guarantee of office space, and an assistant professor of medicine said, "I did not negotiate for parking, and I then found out that it was critical!"

But generally, in this seller's market, both negotiators and non-negotiators among the junior faculty were reasonably well satisfied with the arrangements they had made, as in these examples from surgery and medicine:

> Salary and benefits were fine. The only issue I pushed at the time was to be in control of the hand service.
>
> There wasn't really much to negotiate. They said, what do you think you need, and I gave them a list, and they said, oh, is that all. I have no clinical responsibilities this year and will have three months next year.

Senior faculty members stressed independence as they talked about the final job negotiations; there was a strong pattern of desire for autonomy, as in these comments:

> Very important was my own inpatient ward, my own unit with my own house staff. That was sort of a sticking point.

> Authority to run the center, a computer here and at home, an office of my own.

> Autonomy. I almost took a job someplace else. Ultimately I wrote a letter stating x, y, z, and if not, forget it, and they accepted it.

> Essentially I negotiated space and staff, technical professional support, and the freedom to hire and fire. I made it clear that I was going to run the place the way I wanted to, and I didn't want any interference.

Space was mentioned by almost everyone interviewed, and all of the facilities I visited showed signs of construction—including creative internal renovations where external expansion was restricted. The need was summed up by a professor of pediatrics in this way:

> Space is a major problem, and we couldn't reach a final solution, but it required a lot of talking. I met with several other heads in the hospital. If you have uncovered a formula for that, put it in your book. [Unfortunately, I have not.]

FITTING IN

As the chief of cardiology quoted at the end of chapter 3 averred, not all clinical science appointments are successful. By the time I had arrived on the scene to interview the faculty members appointed in the previous year, several had decided they did not "fit in." Eight assistant professors had left—situated in four schools and in the specialties of radiology (three), surgery (two), anesthesia, medicine, and neurology (one in each). Two of the radiologists had moved on to other academic jobs, one to private practice; the surgeons had opted for private practice and a health maintenance organization; the internist had joined a private hospital staff; and the neurologist had taken another academic job. At a prestigious academic medical center in the East, a coveted professor of medicine had decamped to his former university; the chairman characterized his departure in this way:

> After the early interviews we decided that he was the one. But he was here eight months, and he antagonized everybody. We couldn't get his lab built as rapidly as possible because of an

asbestos problem, and he got very impatient about that. It just didn't work out.

Of the 168 appointees who were interviewed, three (all assistant professors) informed me during interviews that they were looking for another job: a psychiatrist, specifically recruited, who had been asked to leave for what sounded like political reasons; and two radiologists, who were seeking private-practice situations. One of the radiologists, who also had been a specific recruitment, directed me to a recent journal article decrying the condition of academic radiology, and added:

> Everybody's leaving academic radiology; it's falling apart. Chairmen are into self-aggrandizement. The clinical is pushed. If all you're going to do is see patients, you might as well be in private practice making money.

Another thirteen assistant professors expressed feelings of ambivalence, ranging from, "There is this thing about the red dress; you wear it one day and you like it, and the next time you wear it, you don't," to "I took an academic position to prepare for boards and to finish a book I'm writing, but I will not stay in academic medicine for more than five years." And there was this complaint from an assistant professor based at a hospital affiliated with a medical school separated from its main campus:

> The [academic] title is important to me because it's a reminder that I'm an academic. Unfortunately, it's a political arrangement here. I don't feel like I'm a faculty member of a medical school. I very much appreciate being a part of it, and I certainly teach and produce enough to earn the title, but I miss having the rest of the campus across the street. I'd like to go to the faculty lounge and meet people who teach history and law and music. I will probably leave in two or three years because I do want to be part of a university.

All but two of the relatively disgruntled thirteen assistant professors had chosen the job over other opportunities; the two who had not were residents who had stayed on. (In fact, among the total 133 junior faculty members interviewed, more than one-fourth had not considered any other jobs; about half of those had been residents or fellows who had joined the faculty.)

After this sorting took place, there were 152 new faculty members (at all ranks) who presented themselves as reasonably satisfied with their positions—not a bad ratio, suggesting that the matchings in this study represented a good fit for the organization.

The other piece of the fit was provided by chairs in their assessment of the new faculty members. About the senior appointees, as might be expected, the chairs were uniformly positive. The question asked was whether or not the appointment would have a long-run effect on the program, and the answers included these, about a professor and an associate professor:

> Yes. There is unquestionably a growth factor associated with her division. It will have an overall impact on the direction of the hospital; the development of transplant programs will have a major impact.
>
> Yes, and a short-run effect too, which is more important from my standpoint because I don't expect to be chairman much longer. Medical schools have long-range plans but they are sometimes a year or a year and a half the way things are going.

More surprising was chair reaction to junior appointments—highly positive, with the exception of eight less sanguine statements, of which this was typical: "She will make an outstanding contribution for five years, and then there will be a question. This is typical of young faculty members in schools of medicine today."

But the majority of comments about assistant professors were laudatory. These constitute a sample from each of the six schools:

> Yeah, I am delighted to have her! There is a deficiency in my department in research; I need to build. When I came here there was not a single NIH grant in the department. I would consider making her chief of the division in another couple of years.
>
> I sure do! I think he's really quite good. In a very short time he has had a stimulating effect on our laboratory, pushing people a little bit—new ideas.
>
> Yes, I think he's already established himself as a key member of the group. He is very stable and a collaborative type of individual, which you need in complex programs. It is very important because the group tends not to collaborate very well.

> Yeah! He has got tremendously good people management techniques. He is a born politician who can get things done, and he knows how to deal with people. He has good administrative talents. I'm thinking about making him residency director in the next three or four years—maybe chief of obstetrics someday.

> Again, her personality has already had a significant impact because she seems to be unaffected by a lot of the trivia that the rest of us are bothered by. She just goes on and does her job and does it extremely well. She has had tremendous impact psychologically.

> Oh, yeah! It's already added a new area of expertise that this division didn't have and that the department over the past several years has been trying to acquire—molecular technique.

Summing up, this chapter has reviewed the study data for insights into the choices made in academic medicine, with these findings: The recruits in the pool for academic jobs chose the medical profession early and became attracted to academics primarily through their interest in teaching and research. The organization selecting them behaved in a somewhat more democratic fashion than was the case in earlier stages of recruitment. Departments selected candidates subjectively, assessing their research, clinical, and teaching abilities—and, in the case of senior people, management skills. Junior candidates, similarly, were attracted to the specific job by research opportunities—but more so by the geographic location of the job, which might include accommodation of personal relationships. Senior candidates were anxious to display their management skills in an autonomous manner. Choices at all levels were influenced by family considerations, but not substantially by salary. The large majority of new faculty members were pleased with their decisions, and chairs expressed confidence in the hiring choices they had made.

But this best of all possible worlds is a highly competitive labor market, and a major concern revealed in the study was represented by this comment from a chairman of radiology about a new assistant professor: "The only concern I have about him is that I'm not sure he'll be here that long. Several departments have tried to recruit him already."

Chapter 5

Leaving the Clinical Science Department

> I just didn't fit in. There was departmental instability; I was unable to develop programs; I had no input in decisions affecting me. There was an excess time and effort demand—clinical, teaching, research.
>
> Assistant Professor of Psychiatry

> I was very happy there. It was just the perfect job elsewhere.
>
> Assistant Professor of Surgery

Whether a case of not "fitting in" at the old job or the "perfect job" somewhere else, the employment situation apparently became problematic for a number of faculty members in the study sample, leading them to exit from the medical school. In the academic year 1986–1987, the fifty departments with terminations lost 149 faculty members in thirteen specialties and in all academic ranks (Table 5.1).

The volume of terminations, similar to that of appointments, was heaviest in the larger specialties of internal medicine, pediatrics, obstetrics and gynecology, and surgery—but not in radiology, in spite of concerns that had been expressed about turnover in that specialty. Also, like appointments, the majority of terminations were from assistant professor and tenure-track positions.

Incidentally, the widespread belief among nonmedical faculty members that medical school faculty turnover is high compared to the arts

Table 5.1
Terminations

Specialty Group/ Specialty	Tenured or Tenure Track Inst/ Assoc	Asst Prof	Assoc Prof	Prof	Not Tenure Track Inst/ Assoc	Asst Prof	Assoc Prof	Prof	Total
Medical									
Dermatology		1	1	2					4
Family Medicine			1			1	1		3
Medicine	1	10	6	9	1	8		1	36
Neurology		3		1					4
Pediatrics		7	2			3	2		14
Total	1	21	10	12	1	12	3	1	61
Surgical									
Ob-Gyn		8		3	1	1			13
Ophthalmology		2				1			3
Otolaryngology		1	1						2
Surgery		3	2	7		2	4		18
Total		14	3	10	1	4	4		36
Behavioral									
Psychiatry		13	1	3	1	3	2		23
Total		13	1	3	1	3	2		23
Hospital-based									
Anesthesia		4	3	1	1	1			10
Pathology		3	2	2		4	1		12
Radiology		4				3			7
Total		11	5	3	1	8	1		29
All	1	59	19	28	4	27	10	1	149

and sciences was not supported by these figures. The 149 terminations from a total population of 4,311 faculty members in the clinical science departments in this study compared favorably to the 167 out of 3,302 in my arts and sciences study.

The terminations noted in Table 5.1 included only three deaths; thus, there were 146 faculty members who ostensibly departed. However, fifteen of those were retirees, and a most interesting feature of the retirement of a medical faculty member was that it might not really occur. Eleven of the fifteen were still at work in the department; about one, a chair said, "He is not doing anything different from what he was before." These were other comments:

> He is an extremely active member of the faculty. We pay for a secretary for him, and he administers some of our educational programs. The students like him.

> She's in and out doing projects for us, is now working on the annual report. She comes to grand rounds every week. She is very helpful because she knows a lot of things about the department and the school.

So, eliminating the retirees, who may or may not have left, there were 131 faculty members who moved from one job to another. How, why, and where they moved, and what effect their move had on the department they left—and on them—are the subjects examined in this chapter.

CIRCUMSTANCES OF DEPARTURE

The departing group of faculty members included twenty Ph.D.s, most of whom moved on to academic positions elsewhere. A few were in one- or two-year "advanced training" positions or lost their nontenure track jobs in budget cuts or reorganizations but most moved voluntarily.

The 111 M.D.s were a more diverse group, although most resigned voluntarily, and more than half moved to academic jobs (Table 5.2).

About one-third of the group (36 out of 111, or 32.4 percent) defected to private practice. Again the number and proportion leaving academic medicine compares favorably to the number and proportion in my arts and sciences study who left higher education (39 out of 124, or 31.5 percent).

The choice of private practice was stratified by school ranking, with less than 20 percent of the faculty members departing from top-ranked schools going into private practice, but with 52 percent of those leaving lower-ranked schools doing so. The pattern was further skewed by a

Table 5.2
Destination of Departing M.D.s

Destination	From Schools Ranked in Top 19		From Schools Ranked 20 to 50		Total	
	No.	%	No.	%	No.	%
Academic job	39	60.0	20	43.5	59	53.2
Private practice	12	18.5	24	52.2	36	32.4
Other	10	15.4	2	4.3	12	10.8
Unknown	4	6.1			4	3.6
Total	65	100.0	46	100.0	111	100.0

preponderance of such movements in the lowest-ranked school, where nineteen out of the twenty-three departing M.D.s chose private practice. Differentiation was also an effect of rank: 36 percent of the departing junior faculty members, but only 24 percent of the senior members, elected private practice.

The exodus from the lowest-ranked medical school appeared to be precipitated by a new administration, which raised academic standards. These termination actions were classified by the school as voluntary resignations, but many were clearly compelled by organizational changes. Comments about the former colleagues were typified by these from chairmen of psychiatry and pathology: "I inherited him; he has gone into private practice," and "He simply did not want to go through the academic rigors."

In fact, there were only five acknowledged instances of tenure or reappointment denial in the total sample, taking place at only two schools. (These were all departmental, rather than institutional, decisions.) There were, however, a few references to academic stress in chair responses, leading to the conclusion that at least some of the resignations characterized as voluntary were marginally so. These were representative comments:

> He left to work for a for-profit private psychiatric hospital. He was concerned that because I am avowedly a more academic chair than my predecessor, I might value him less.
>
> He was not put up for promotion; it was a decision of the promotions committee within the department. He had requested promotion a year early, and there had been a lot of discussions with him. There were also some personal interaction problems with other people on the staff. The decision was really his—it was presented in a way as his decision to look for something else.
>
> He knew from me that at his current rate of scientific productivity, at his rate of progress, he would not achieve tenure. I think he would have been incapable of accelerating that rate. He was not in an area that I could help him with.

Even where a truly voluntary move was to occur, and where the department regretted the impending loss, few efforts were made to retain the junior faculty member. Chairs generally explained their reluctance to attempt intervention in terms of the uselessness of the effort, as in these remarks:

> When people want to go into private practice, we have no chance of keeping them. Once they've turned their head in that direction, there is no turning back.
>
> Once individuals have come to that point—of making a qualitative choice—there is not a great deal you can do.

There is also the ever-present pressure to have a self-supporting department composed of self-supporting faculty members that might preclude retention efforts, as in this case: "We didn't have the money to keep him. He wasn't generating grant support."

There was somewhat more retention effort exerted for senior faculty members, although frequently there was ambivalence expressed as well. The mixed feelings were expressed by chairmen in these two examples:

> We gave him more personnel, flexibility with his own time. But in truth this was a good job for him. It would have been a mistake for him not to take it.
>
> Yes, we tried to keep him, but it was a very good opportunity for him.

These rather half-hearted motions were balanced by strong feelings and efforts in a few cases. In both of the following situations, the pull to the new job was just too strong:

> He and I collaborated in our research, and I asked him if getting him a larger lab would help. He was candid, said he didn't think so, that he wanted a chance to run his own show.
>
> I nearly cut his legs off. I was close on salary—he said he wasn't leaving for money.

Generally, there is a feeling of mobility conveyed about academic medicine (although the faculties in this study were a fairly stable group)—one young faculty member had remarked, "You always have to be jockeying for position, thinking about your next job." And although one chairman remarked that he would like to build a department that no one would ever leave, he characterized his idea as something of a fantasy.

FINDING THE NEW JOB

The departing junior faculty members—even those who had left not quite voluntarily—were not facing unemployment. Following the pattern revealed in earlier chapters, investigation into the movement of these faculty members leaving a job showed the same particularized recruitment. One assistant professor of psychiatry said that he had located his new job through an ad, but the remainder of the respondents mentioned personal contacts—one said flatly, "old boy network."

Chairs describing a departure provided the following accounts: "The new chair there knew him, thought highly of him"; "he got to know them on a sabbatical"; "they were rebuilding a department and recruited him." Again, the inevitability of movement was reflected in this contention of a chairman of radiology: "Our good people are recruited constantly."

The chairs' observations were matched by explanations from faculty members who had left:

> I was recruited vigorously over a two-year period (they sought me out).
>
> I was recruited by my old chairman (from fellowship days).
>
> I wasn't looking around. This was the only job I looked at during my time there. The chairman here called me up and offered the job to me on the phone; he is a nephrologist and knew me somewhat from that. My former chief was with him [the chairman] for fifteen years or so—including M.D. and residency.

Accommodation for spouse employment figured in the termination sample as it had in appointments. An assistant professor of pediatrics gave this illustration of the facilitation of her recruitment:

> My husband and I were both looking for jobs. My husband met his present boss at a meeting, and this man scouted out my department here to see if there were anything for me—he really wanted my husband.

Consistent with the reluctance to make other than rudimentary efforts to keep faculty members, chairs frequently took active steps to encourage the promotion of a faculty member through outside recruitment. As one explained:

> A number of us are fairly prominent nationally and are able to promote others in national positions. We helped him get prominent posts, and he attracted attention.

In a similar situation, a chairman of medicine talked about supporting a professor in his department for a position as division chief elsewhere:

> The chairman of the department there was formerly in my department before I came here, and he called me and asked me if I could recommend somebody, and I recommended [the professor who had left]. They hit it off, and he hired him. He has written to me that he is very pleased with his choice.

More general comments were these: "He had received a series of written inquiries to come look at this job or that job"; "they've given him an offer once a month"; "he was very well known—had three chair offers simultaneously." And about a professor who had assumed a prestigious national position, a chairman of surgery accentuated the importance of support from prominent people in academic medicine by saying that the appointment had been facilitated by a distinguished chairman whom he described as the "kingmaker."

There were no surprises as the personal contact nature of recruitment was repeated in responses from senior faculty members who had changed jobs. These were typical statements from former associate professors:

> I was told of it by the chief in my field at my current place of work, at a "chat" at a national meeting.
>
> Personal contact from my lecturing at the new facility.
>
> My chairman became the dean at the new institution and asked me to come with him.

COMPARING OLD AND NEW JOBS

One might expect that moving to a new faculty job would entail an improvement in the faculty member's position, and this indeed was the case. The fifty-nine M.D. faculty members who were known to have left to take other academic jobs generally maintained or improved their rank and salary position, with only a few exceptions (Table 5.3).

Thirty-one of the faculty members (53 percent of the total) achieved higher academic rank or responsibility in the move; the proportion was

Table 5.3
New Academic Job, by Characteristics

Characteristic of New Job	Number of Faculty Members: Moving from Schools Ranked 1 to 19		Moving from Schools Ranked 20 to 50		
	Junior	Senior	Junior	Senior	Total
Academic Rank					
Same	11	1	4	5	21
Higher*	12	12	3	4	31
Unknown	3		4		7
Total	26	13	11	9	59
Salary					
Lower			1		1
Same	4	2	1	2	9
Higher	15	9	5	6	35
Unknown	7	2	4	1	14
Total	26	13	11	9	59
School Ranking					
1 to 19	9	2	2	1	14
20 to 50	8	4	3	4	19
Below 50	6	7	3	3	19
Not ranked or unknown	3		3	1	7
Total	26	13	11	9	59

*In the case of senior faculty members who moved, the "higher academic rank" category includes prestige or authority added to the rank of full professor previously held.

73 percent at the senior level. Salary increases were obtained by 59 percent of the total sample (68 percent of the senior faculty).

Again, as in the recruitment portion of the study, the notion of movement within a school's reputational ranking group is not well supported. Almost three-quarters of the faculty members who left positions at the top-ranked schools in the study moved to schools ranked 20 or below, with one-third moving to schools ranked below 50 (this last group including a majority of the departing senior faculty). On the other hand, only one-fifth of the faculty members leaving schools ranked 20 to 50 moved down in the rankings—and three moved up to a top-nineteen school.

Perhaps the factor in these movements that is most clearly defined in the interview data is that the best opportunity, or running one's own show, may not be available at a top crowded with avid researchers. Instead, the opportunity may exist at a school that has a lower prestige rating and is looking for people who will enhance its image (i.e., people from schools perceived to enjoy more prestige). Further, those schools that were recruiting from the top nineteen apparently had amassed resources to support a level and mix of activity that offered greater opportunity, or at least the perception of greater opportunity, to the departing faculty member.

Along with the comparisons of academic rank and salary, senior faculty members who moved to lower-ranked schools had these comments to make about the power they could wield in their new positions:

> I play a greater role in shaping the department [as vice chairman]. The opportunity to do research is greater because I have protected time.
>
> I have more influence since I am now division director. Opportunities are increased since more local funds to support research are available.
>
> I have 80 percent research time with few clinical responsibilities! Excellent academic opportunities. Better travel and computer support.

In similar terms, a chairman lamenting a departure may have exaggerated, but probably not much, when he said, "They gave him the world; he is really a superstar. He got ten faculty positions and 12,000 square feet of space. His will be one of the premier departments."

A full professor who had made an essentially lateral institutional move touched on the same point of opportunity: "I am much more independent [as chairman], and I have the possibility of expanding and improving an already existing residency program."

Those who left assistant professor positions, too, stressed opportunities, as did this internist who had moved down to a lower-ranked school but up in academic rank and responsibility:

> I ran a research program with one technician in a room about this size [interview took place in medium-sized office]. Here I have sixteen faculty, able to organize their research and guide them, able to develop a broader research program myself by having more space and more money to work with. I am associate professor and chief here in a department that I think is outstanding—a lot of resources available here.

Several junior people who had moved laterally or downward (institutionally) mentioned greater opportunities for research in comparing their new job with the old one, in references like these: "Improved clinical research opportunities"; "a great cardiology colleague to work with in my research"; "independent laboratory, protected time, excellent opportunities."

The phenomenon of the move "down" but "up" is typified by the description of the move of an M.D.-Ph.D. assistant professor, who could be expected to have specialized research interests and skills, from a top-five school to one ranked below fifty. His former chairman commented as follows:

> His rank and salary are higher—twice the salary he was making here. There is even more emphasis on research. He is director of a research lab with minimal service and teaching responsibilities. His interests are very closely allied to the new chair there—experimental toxicology—there are very few of them in the world.

PUSHING AND PULLING

There are generally acknowledged to be push and pull factors in any job change—confirmed in this study by the appointment data—although for professionals the pull to a new situation is frequently stronger than the push from the old one. The pull for the fifty-two respondents in this study was closely comparable to the reasons that new appointees had given for taking their positions (Table 5.4).

A difference from the appointee sample was the preponderance of promotion alone as an attraction—given as the first reason by more than one-quarter of all respondents and more than 60 percent of the senior respondents. The promotion was linked to other reasons, but it was clearly first. Following are examples of new chairs or division chiefs elaborating on their choices:

> To be chief of gastroenterology. Second, they offered all that I asked for to create a GI [gastrointestinal] section. And I was given a significant amount of funds to increase my research efforts.

> Besides the opportunity to become division chief, I had the opportunity to advance my research through collaboration at the new institution.

> I came to [new institution] as division chief in pulmonary medicine—ability to be chief of the division. The second thing was

Table 5.4
Reasons for Choosing New Job

Reason Given by Faculty Member	Moving from Junior Faculty to: Academic Position	Moving from Junior Faculty to: Private Practice	Moving from Senior Faculty to: Academic Position	Moving from Senior Faculty to: Private Practice	Moving from Senior Faculty to: Other	Total No.	Total %
Promotion	3		11			14	26.9
Research opportunities	3	1	1	1		6	11.5
Geographic location	2	2	1			5	9.6
Opportunity to build or develop department or program	2		3			5	9.6
Academic/clinical balance	4					4	7.7
Respect/liking for colleagues in new department	4					4	7.7
Independence		2		1		3	5.8
Respect/liking for individual who recruited	2					2	3.8
Money		1	1			2	3.8
Other	1	2	1	3		7	13.6
Total	21	8	18	1	4	52	100.0

that there were new and larger possibilities for collaboration in my investigative interests.

Research opportunities similar to those already noted were the first cause of taking the new job in the next largest group of respondents, slightly more than 10 percent. An assistant professor, whose academic contract had not been renewed (because he did not have grant funds) and who had gone into private practice (he hoped temporarily), recognized that for him the push was stronger. Still, he was able to characterize a pull to his current situation in this way, "It gave me the opportunity to develop new research directives—to change from fundamental to applied clinical research."

A former associate professor, a Ph.D., who had left a department of surgery to move with an M.D. colleague to a private hospital, characterized the previous job as one where "research [was] in the rear of the bus," and cited these pull factors to the new job:

> Opportunities for research—strong philosophic and financial commitment by new facility to support research; good research facilities with expansion under way; major clinical resources; wide variety of new colleagues with primary research interests, plus opportunities for interaction with other disciplines.

And another associate professor, who had moved to a new academic position at the same rank and salary, was pulled by the "opportunity to do research" having found that in his previous position he had "too many clinical and administrative responsibilities and unclear hopes that the future would be better."

The reasons of geographic location and the opportunity to build or develop a department or program that were the most prevalent first choices, respectively, of junior and senior appointees appeared on the list of attractions for departed faculty members as well. In addition, as remarked on earlier, spouse employment was a positive factor in several moves, although not the first choice for any respondent.

A new entry here was money, which had not been mentioned as a top reason by any appointee. Salary was a pull factor for a psychiatrist who went into private practice and an otolaryngologist who moved to another academic position (both leaving the lowest ranked medical school in the sample). For the psychiatrist, research was a factor as well, but in this instance, negative. He wrote that in his former job he had "no time for research and no guidance for research by senior faculty" amid "unrealistic expectations for research" and so was pulled by "salary," but also to "continue my teaching efforts" and have "no research requirement."

A second entry was independence—a pull factor for three former faculty members who left to go into private practice. One of them, an M.D.-Ph.D. psychiatrist who had left one of the top-ranked schools to join a group practice, wrote about her preference in these words:

> Self-employed. More control of time. More opportunities, including research opportunities. Absence of hassle. Greater ability to get support for initiatives. More broadening clinical responsibility. Very good continuing medical education.

Although the pull to a new position might be stronger than the push from the old in most cases, conditions at the former job appeared to have had an influence on the move, especially with respect to the organizational culture (Table 5.5).

The primary push factors were described—again in terms comparable to those used by new appointees—as organizational change or conflict or an environment in which the faculty member had limited professional opportunities. Organizational issues were cited by both junior and senior faculty as major reasons for leaving. One assistant professor of anesthesia who had moved at the same rank wrote these complaints about the job she had left:

> (1) Frustrations with chairman—dishonesty, inability to accomplish necessary changes; (2) lack of teaching; (3) lack of communication with surgeons, inability to manage anesthetic due to preconceived, set in concrete rules by surgeons.

Table 5.5
Reasons for Leaving Old Job

Reason Given by Faculty Member	Moving from Junior Faculty to		Moving from Senior Faculty to			Total	
	Academic Position	Private Practice	Academic Position	Private Practice	Other	No.	%
Organizational change, conflict	8		5		2	15	28.9
Stagnant, no opportunity to advance	2	2	7			11	21.2
Lack of research opportunities	4		1			5	9.6
High stress, not in control	2	1	2			5	9.6
Lack of support	1	1	1			3	5.8
No balance, too much clinical	2					2	3.8
Family reasons		2		1		3	5.8
Geographic location	2					2	3.8
Had accomplished everything I could					2	2	3.8
Other		2	2			4	7.7
Total	21	8	18	1	4	52	100.0

A former assistant professor of medicine who had moved to the position of division chief and rank of associate professor talked about leaving in this way:

> It was 99 percent pull. I was content there, but it was clear that I could not expand my research program. There were too many people there near me and if I had moved into other research areas it would have made them angry. I would not have moved for an equal position, but I do like some things better about this department—this department tries to balance out the clinical-teaching needs with the research needs. I have been able to establish a clinical program and teaching program, both of which I enjoy a lot—there is no reward for that there.

Senior respondents were more likely to cite problems such as the "political situation between the University and the V.A." More personal disagreements were mentioned by a few, as by this former associate professor who had moved up to chairwoman and full professor: "I couldn't stand my chairman or division chief. I thought they were arbitrary and made irrational decisions."

Similar sentiments were expressed in more measured tones by this professor of surgery:

> (1) The lack of support for research, teaching, and administration, especially since I had been acting chairman for two years. (2) I had some dissatisfaction/disagreement with the new chairman's decisions related to decentralization of the department.

A stagnant or no-growth environment—a kind of professional limbo—was listed as the most important push factor by a number of respondents. The following quotes came from an assistant professor who moved at the same rank to the school where he had completed his fellowship and an associate professor who had moved to chair and full professor:

> Felt division was stagnant; 100 percent time clinical with no time for research, yet expectation within university was for research even though not in any way supported by new division chief. After seven to eight months I decided to leave.

> Professionally I guess it was the "pull" factors. The only reasons I was thinking of leaving were that I was where I was going to be, section chief—there was nowhere to go.

The reasons given by medical faculty members for leaving (except for the references to clinical work) were remarkably like those given for faculty members in the arts and sciences. For example, a colleague had said about a departed faculty member in the arts and sciences, "There was personal tension between him and the local star in the field." The medical counterpart of that statement came from a member of the department of medicine, who said, "There was a more prominent lab run by a more senior faculty member here who had trained him." Even the oddity was replicated. In a locale of high property values, an associate professor in the arts and sciences had left in this way: "He gave notice one week before the end of the semester. He made a killing in real estate and said to hell with it."

The medical outlier was also an associate professor who, according to his former chairman, had engineered a similar career change:

> He is a multi-millionaire—an appointment made in this department many, many years ago, and he never did anything in the department that I could determine. He worked over in the hospital and did a lot of leukemia research. When his grant went off, he went dry. He said he'd like to take a year off and see if he liked farming better than he did this, and he did, and so he resigned.

Overall, there was not a great degree of consistency in a comparison of chairs' perceptions and faculty members' reports of leaving. Less than half of the chairs gave the same reasons for either the attraction of the new job or the impetus to leave the old one that were given by junior faculty members. Their batting average was better—slightly more than half—at agreement with senior faculty members on what they liked about the new position, but poor on reasons for leaving. Where the chair had pinpointed family concerns: "Well, I think there was a matter of lifestyle. They had just had a child and wanted to move into a better environment." The former associate professor of psychiatry gave these as his major reasons for leaving: "(1) Lack of support for my work; (2) lack of support for program I developed; (3) poor administration."

About one-fourth of the chairs said simply "I don't know" or "I'm not sure" when asked about either the push or pull factors in a junior departure. Beyond that, they expressed a rather strong belief that there was no push—it was all pull. Where they did offer other opinions, no new factors emerged, but the emphasis was somewhat different. For example, where a junior faculty member had reported that he left primarily because of stress in the job, that his "areas of research were not proceeding as rapidly as I desired," his chairman said:

> I would have been very pleased with him, and he would have been very happy here, but his wife just didn't like it here and didn't want to bring up their kids here. There was too much crime. But he didn't want to be any other place than a big city.

Especially illuminating were the following two illustrations from a top-ranked school and a lower-ranked school. In the first case, the chairman said:

> He was developing quite well. He got an outside foundation fellowship at a reasonably senior level, felt he was being overwhelmed and unsupported and went to another academic job in the city. I thought it would not work out that well, and he is now discovering that, but is still working at it.

The assistant professor in question had a different viewpoint:

> The chairman was hostile and threatened by my success and my opinion being taken over his at times; when I received a private grant, which gave me more independence as a junior faculty person, he told me I would not only have a salary cut but had to give up private practice earnings to the department for the next three years ($90,000 income) although I documented the Foundation allowed me to practice.

Further, the junior respondent showed no signs of disenchantment with his new position, and, in fact, referred to it in these terms: "Better atmosphere of department; better future opportunity; better salary; better practice arrangement; more learning for me." From the lower-ranked school, the chairman said, "She had personal problems. She was a very poor teacher, got the worst student evaluations."

The assistant professor who had moved at the same academic rank to a higher-rated school wrote, "Could not tolerate department chairman—'son of a bitch,' " and had this to say about her new situation, "Better school, better department. Better overall quality of students, residents.

More cohesive faculty. Much more of the Harvard tradition in which I was trained."

Either these chairs had little rapport with the faculty members who had left, or time had blunted memory, or they were reluctant to be candid on the subject. At any rate, the respondent groups were frequently seen to be inhabiting different worlds.

An interesting footnote to the push–pull discussion is the statement from four of the nine termination respondents who had gone into private practice that they had intended to stay in academic medicine when they took the job they had left. (The other five said they had been "undecided," or it was "questionable," or they were undertaking a "trial period.") Among the group that had moved to other academic positions, there was little ambivalence, expressed by only three persons. To the question as to intent to stay in academic medicine, one said, "Yes, if I could support my family," and apparently found that he could. Another said he was "not positive" and had "planned three to ten years with a career decision at that time," which turned out to favor academic medicine. The third, who had moved to a chairmanship, wrote this response:

> My intent when I first went on the faculty there was to determine if I liked academic medicine, and if I did, I would remain. I found that I enjoyed academics and thus remained on the full-time faculty for twenty-three years, rising from instructor in surgery to professor of surgery and, eventually, acting chairman of the department of surgery for two and a half years, and then remained on the staff for an additional ten years as professor of surgery.

ASSESSING EFFECTS

There are two basic questions about the effect of these terminations: (1) Is the faculty member satisfied with his or her new position? (2) What was the impact on the clinical science department that suffered the loss?

On the first point, chairs were about evenly divided between "yes" and "I don't know" when asked about the former faculty member's current job satisfaction. There were only two exceptions to that pattern. About a former assistant professor who had moved within the top-fifteen group of schools, the chairman said, "No, and that's a shame. Maybe he's one of those poor souls who will never be content."

(I was reminded of the academic gadfly noted in the arts and sciences study—"always on the market.")

The other exception was the assistant professor who had left to run a service at a for-profit psychiatric hospital. In that case, the chairman's comment was this: "He wants to come back. He misses the area, and he feels that he has done what he can and wants to come back to the university. We are trying to work something out for him. (He is making a lot more money there.)"

With respect to the "don't knows," the following was an interesting comment from the academic about the private practitioner: "I don't know. These people just drop out of sight—it is the end of their visible career." A "yes" was accompanied by a reminder of what a small world academic medicine is: "He is coming back for our second alumni reunion next week and will be a speaker at a symposium we're running."

All but two of the responding faculty members (and not the same two individuals already noted) answered "yes" to the job satisfaction question, some adding "extremely" or "very much." The dissidents were assistant professors who had gone into private practice (one after denial of reappointment); both were searching for new academic jobs. In addition, an associate professor had rather ambivalent feelings: "Yes and no. I miss my friends and some of the roles I formerly played." A professor concurred: "Yes—except my former institution had more prestige."

The roles played by a faculty member were apparently important in considering the impact of a departure on the department. Perceptions of role varied between chair and faculty member, however, as perceptions had varied between chair and faculty member on the subject of the latter's satisfaction with the new job. Of the fifty-two termination responses that could be compared, there was agreement between chair and former faculty member in only eighteen instances—about a third—and half of those eighteen were senior terminations. Five of the assistant professors who had left agreed realistically that their departure had not made much difference to the department—they wrote comments such as these: "My position was filled in a fairly short time by an equally qualified person," and "replacement physician had similar research interests."

And in a different situation, where her chairwoman had been noncommittal, an assistant professor wrote this about the change her departure might have made in her previous department:

> I think so, although none of the supervisory faculty said so. I ran the pediatric neurology clinic each Friday, and supervised it weekly (which freed up all but one other division member), saw the newborns with neuro problems daily, and did general peds

> sectional attending, and attended morning report daily. Many of the peds residents said they'd miss my teaching. There was *no* response to my letter of resignation. I certainly would have preferred some comment (even if insincere) that I would be missed.

But, of course, it is the opinion of those who survived the departure that matters most in assessing the effect of the departure. Overall, chairs said that the departure of a junior faculty member had made a real change in the department in less than 20 percent of the terminations. Assistant professors were generally viewed by chairs as replaceable parts; they "kept a resident to take his place," or "a fellow helped tide us over," or, most telling, "No, he was at the assistant professor level." (These were the same chairs who had told me how important their new junior appointees were to the department!)

Senior people fared somewhat better, their departures having made a real change in the department in about 50 percent of the terminations. In one of the cases where both parties agreed, the former faculty member wrote that "one of the other centers in the city, to quote its chief, a friend of mine, 'has benefited greatly by my leaving' "; his former chairman said:

> It was a loss of a senior clinical person who left a void that's just gradually being filled in by others, and it meant a loss of a certain dimension within the laboratory research program that he was conducting. He was replaced in part, but you can't really replace someone at that stage in his career.

Subspecialization was a significant factor in the impact of the departure in several cases, as a chairman of pediatrics pointed out: "He was very valuable; there are not many people like him. We could not find a second or third coagulationist—they do not exist."

Although that former faculty member had written in agreement, worth apparently was not always recognized—or perhaps communicated. In several cases, the faculty member had indicated that his departure had made no real difference, but the chairs responded otherwise, as in these examples:

> It left a real void in cardiac surgery—the program fell apart when he left.

> It was a real change because his main strength was his practical approach to patient care from his years of experience. He was an

excellent teacher in a nonthreatening way. He was patient with the residents, able to sit and let them expound on what they thought without blowing his top when they were wrong—he was good at a number of procedures done in family practice and in teaching them those. The residents thought of him as a senior mentor. So yes, we've seen a real change that I'm not very happy with, nor are the residents.

CLASSIFYING MOTIVATION

Since Gouldner (1957) introduced the idea of faculty orientation in liberal arts colleges as being divided into locals and cosmopolitans, and Caplow and McGee (1958) extended the theory to research universities, there have been several attempts to classify faculty members in one of those two categories. The local orientation implied longevity in a particular institution; the cosmopolitan was more likely to move. Later research has suggested a more complex typology, with such factors as age and career stage entering the picture, as well as a growing tendency in America to stay put.

Perhaps because of the structural ambiguity of medical schools, the patterns so far developed do not serve academic medicine. According to Gouldner, locals think of themselves in terms of the institution, and cosmopolitans identify with disciplines. In the environment of academic medicine, *all* faculty members identify with their specialties. All of the faculty members in this sample who had left their jobs belonged to national associations in their specialties and thought of themselves primarily as members of the specialties in which they were certified—as pediatricians, psychiatrists, internists, or family practitioners.

Another part of the test, according to Caplow and McGee, was whether or not those who left were well known professionally outside the institution, with the presumption that those faculty members who left would fit the profile of being well known. Only a third of the departing faculty members in this sample were well known outside the institution.

Where the division in this study occurred was between those faculty members who left to take other academic jobs and those who left to enter private practice. Consider the following:

- One-fifth of all faculty members who left were well known outside the institution.
- One-half of all senior faculty members who left were well known outside the institution.

- One-third of all faculty members moving to academic jobs were well known outside the institution.
- More than one-half of senior faculty members moving to academic jobs were well known outside the institution.

But, only one faculty member who left to enter private practice was well known outside the institution.

Therefore, in the medical faculty the cosmopolitan–local dichotomy is not the appropriate framework for classifying the mobile faculty member. Rather, it is the local, who is not well known outside the institution, who leaves academic medicine. The cosmopolitan may stay in the institution in his or her academic position or move on to another academic position. Thus, the local–cosmopolitan typology is meaningless in terms of medical faculty mobility.

In another approach to the motivation to depart, it has been considered that professional collaboration within the department or institution could be a factor tending to hold the faculty member in position. Again, the experience in the sample did not support the notion. But also again, there was a difference along the dimension of destination. Only one-quarter of the faculty members leaving to enter private practice had collaborated within their department; only one had collaborated with colleagues outside his department. On the other hand, three-quarters of the faculty members (almost all of the senior people) moving to other academic jobs had collaborated with colleagues both within their department and within the institution outside the department.

The conclusion here, of course, is that being well known and participating in collaboration are both manifestations of a research orientation that, in the medical world, has little to do with the identification with a discipline that has been purported to foster mobility. Rather, the research orientation simply keeps the faculty member in academic medicine, somewhere.

It is the subspecialty that has come to the fore in academic medicine; one of the assistant professors who left for a promotion was described by his former chairman in these words: "Yes, he is very well known, but it is a narrow subspecialty. One of the hot areas he works with is transport of molecules."

A MINI-CASE STUDY

In the mid-1980s the dean of an Ivy League medical school appointed a new chairman to head a large department in the school. The department in question was responsible for running a large clinical service in the medical school's teaching hospital. The financial status of the department (and the hospital) was not the best. Cuts in research funds had affected the financial health of the department; the hospital was experiencing problems endemic to the health care industry today that had, in turn, affected patient care income to the department.

The chairman search had dragged on for a long period of time, creating a high level of uncertainty in the department. In addition, the two top contenders for the chairmanship were the chief (Candidate X) and the associate chief (Candidate Y) of the division that shouldered the major clinical burden for the department.

The two candidates were sufficiently different to give the dean and his appointments committee clear policy options in making their selection. Simply put, Candidate X was viewed as valuing research much more highly than Candidate Y. Candidate Y's strengths would be in development of the clinical program.

The dean appointed Candidate Y as chairman of the department.

The choice of chairman precipitated certain changes in departmental focus. These changes were combined with the aftermath of the stress experienced by members of the department, especially the members of the division that had fielded the two candidates, in the long search for a chairman. The combination produced a trickle-down of choices at other levels in the organization, particularly the choice of leaving.

There were four resignations from the division, including the division chief—leaving only three persons (and a handful of residents) to cover the clinical load. The new chairman was forced to add to his first-year responsibilities that of acting division chief, and naturally assigned high priority to filling the clinical hole.

The chairman's first act was to fill the position of division chief and, not surprisingly, he did so by recruiting someone he knew he could trust. The person he selected had done a residency and fellowship in the department and had been on the faculty some years earlier. The chairman said, "He and I worked together for many years and had a good working relationship. We parted friends and maintained the friendship. I called upon him to come back and help me."

The position of division chief was a step up, prestigewise, for the new incumbent, who was then at a less research-oriented school. But, the chairman added:

> He brings good administrative skills for running a large clinical service, which is what we have. A heavy burden of the teaching in

our specialty falls on this group. We run a busy, active service, there are lots of poor patients, and there is a need to supervise the trainees who serve them. And I wanted to develop the clinical research in that area and tie it to the research division and he has a good track record.

The new division chief took a salary cut in moving, and when asked why he was willing to move, said simply, "My personal relationship with [the chairman]. I worked with him for many years, and he needed help."

Three other new members of the division were appointed, all at the assistant professor level. One was kept from a residency, and two were recruited by the division chief from fellowships at his previous institution. Questions about why they took their jobs were answered in these words:

> [The division chief] said, "There's an opening at [this school] and I'm going there, are you interested in coming," and I said, "Yes." I liked the fact that there were young faculty so I wouldn't be coming into something with a set pattern. I admire [the chairman] very much.

> This department is building, a lot of opportunity to build with the department and division—a new chairman—I thought I could grow with the department and play a vital role in it. (The chairman was my residency director.)

> [I was attracted by] the people, the quality of the faculty, and the research and the medical care. The chairman very strongly influenced me—he is a pretty special person. I had the opportunity here to do the type of work I wanted to do, exactly the kind of job I've been looking for.

All three, when asked why they chose academic medicine, stressed the quality of patient care in an academic medical center (a reason given as primary by only a small minority of the sample of new appointees).

The four faculty members who had left—all of whom had moved to other academic jobs—provided a different perspective. The former division chief, who had moved to a chairmanship, was circumspect. He reported that "minimal" efforts had been made to keep him when he had tendered his resignation and wrote the following as his major reasons for leaving: "New chairperson. Lack of support of department by college and hospital."

An assistant professor who had gone with him provided slightly more information in response to the question about his major reasons for leaving: "In order: (1) Mentor left; I would be working with him at new job; (2) not enough opportunity for academic work, too much clinical; (3) salary."

He also noted that his opportunity for research would be improved at the new job.

The other two faculty members who had left were a dual-career couple interviewed in another part of the country. They, too, reported "minimal" efforts made to keep them when they resigned. A composite of their major reasons for leaving follows:

> We were called about these positions when we weren't looking. In the time interval between when we were called and when we decided to leave, we became progressively more disappointed in the direction the department was taking. [The school], particularly with [the new chairman] and the overall financial status of the hospital and department, was difficult. We weren't getting treated any differently in spite of our grants—they thought Ph.D.s could do research as well as M.D.s. When it looked like [the former division chief] might become chairman there—he valued research—we would have had a mechanism to buy out of a lot of clinical work, sharing a position for six months of the year and going off the malpractice insurance, etc., when we weren't clinical. Besides the lack of the new chairman's interest in research, basically he wanted the M.D.s to earn a lot of clinical dollars, which is not why we went into academic medicine.

The preceding narrative illustrates several facts of life affecting faculty mobility in medical schools today. First, the financial status of the department and the hospital were primary concerns in the selection of a chairman. Second, vacancies forced the new chairman to rely on personal relationship to recruit a new division chief, who in turn was willing to leave a higher paying (but less prestigious) job to come to his friend's aid. Third, the new division chief, facing heavy clinical responsibilities, recruited junior people that he knew personally whose interests were primarily clinical (although this might place them in a minority in the total organization). And finally, articulation of an organizational culture for the department—with an emphasis on clinical work—had prompted resignations of faculty members who were otherwise oriented.

So, the "fitting in" of faculty members may change over time, and the factors involved in leaving the department become an important part of the faculty mobility picture.

Chapter 6

Medical Faculty Mobility: A Conceptual Summary

Dr. Thomas P. Stossel of Harvard Medical School and Massachusetts General Hospital, wrote a rather pessimistic fable in 1987 about the medical school in the year 2007 (Stossel, 1987). In the fable, his protagonist, a medical student who was about to graduate, was awaiting word on her first job, which bore no resemblance in either choice or process to that described in the preceding chapters of this book. By 2007 medical schools had abandoned service and taught only general fundamentals; new M.D.s acquired their clinical skills during subsequent employment. The student would have choices, of course—she hoped to become a junior associate with the prestigious health firm of Lockjaw, Warburton, and Tytesphyncter Medical Research and Providers, Incorporated, subsidiary of Arf Dog Food, Automotive and Medical Enterprises, but she shuddered at the thought of a forced alternative such as Sears Roebuck Research, specializing in drive-in lithotripsy or one of the cut-rate hospitals owned by the insurance risk pool. While waiting out the selection process, the student dipped into a history of American medicine and was astonished to learn that at one time the university and the hospital had joined forces, and that important clinical investigation had taken place *in the medical school*. As Dr. Stossel wrote, "Academic medicine was in the ivory tower and the real world at the same time."

Medical faculty mobility—that is, joining or leaving the academic medical organization—takes place in an environment of contradiction created by this dual role of academic medicine. In retrospect, it seems unfortunate that the service-connected differences of the medical school have not been more thoughtfully appreciated by the larger university, or the academic similarities more carefully integrated. Today, the stress of the medical academician's role is intensified by external pressures being brought to bear on the hospital-based health care system, as well as by internal pressures arising out of the medical school–university relationship.

Thus, the mobility processes of the medical faculty, as indicated in the preceding chapters, bear the imprint of the real world even as they grapple with the norms of the ivory tower. In this last chapter, faculty mobility in Dr. Stossel's medical school of the golden past—the one visited by this study—is viewed through the separate and combined lenses of academia and the hospital.

THE IVORY TOWER

There are a multitude of ways in which the academy makes the medical school its own, and, through the examination of medical faculty mobility in these pages, we have seen much evidence of the ownership. Perhaps the most obvious manifestation is the incorporation in the medical school of elements of the research culture of the university—especially, the growth of academics in a specialty or increased academic expectations of faculty that were mentioned by so many of the respondents. The development of research in the medical school has not only paralleled the acceptance of the German research model in American universities but, in fact, has been in the forefront.

The most critical process for developing and strengthening the research culture is the selection of new faculty members who have a quality training and a commitment to research (Dill, 1986). Most of the selection decisions concerning junior faculty in this study acknowledged that need; successful candidates were described as impressive in "research ability and training" or as "doing very good research" or as having "first-rate training." New faculty members appreciated the "commitment of this department to its junior faculty doing research" or the opportunity "to develop a research program."

Another key to maintaining the research culture is support through institutional policies for a faculty workload that encourages research, reflected in this study by the emphasis on protected time. New junior faculty members negotiated time away from clinical duties for research; chairs presented the notion of critical mass, that is, a sufficient number of faculty members to provide adequate clinical coverage and to allow time for research.

The research culture was also furthered in recruitment through the prestige factor—a majority of the M.D.s appointed had completed residencies at schools that enjoyed a good reputation in graduate medical education. A related indicator was the large number of new appointees who had completed more than one residency, a fellowship, or all of these, pointing to the amount of subspecialization in the sample. At the individual level in the recruitment process, prestige of individuals in a department drew junior faculty in a few cases.

The research culture had its effect on terminations as well. Junior faculty members who had moved without promotion referred to "improved research opportunities" and "protected time" at the new job and "no time for research" at the old job when explaining their decisions to move. And it was clear from the downward drift in senior faculty movement (up in responsibility and authority but down in institutional prestige) that lower-ranked schools were intent on improving their positions in the prestige rankings, which depend primarily on research results.

The research culture encompasses the notion of differentiation that results from professionalization of the academic workforce—that is, in the arts and sciences, individuals who consider themselves "zoologists" or "economists" rather than "faculty members." Professionalization in higher education has fragmented the professoriate in the arts and sciences (Clark, 1966); the same is true of the medical school, in spite of the intertwining and interdependence that is a strong feature of academic medicine. One level of differentiation occurs at the medical specialty, with variances in structure and compensation (e.g., higher-paid specialties emphasizing procedures and lower-paid specialties more concerned with primary care) and with varying degrees of attraction for medical students.

But a more significant agent of differentiation in academic medicine today is subspecialization. Subspecialization bears a large share of the responsibility for the tight labor market and for changes in recruiting procedures caused by the increasing complexity of the medical field. Chairs talked about candidates who were "much more specialized, trained in narrower and narrower areas" and said "now everyone is a subspecialist," and they worried about whether or not candidates "have tracked themselves in a way that fits your needs." Subspecialization, in fact, may fragment a specialty into the "little fiefdoms and little sections," as noted by one respondent, with each fiefdom and section having its advanced residents and fellows. Robert Petersdorf growled in his 1978 paper, "The Doctors' Dilemma," "Directors of subspecialty programs consider it a God-given right to have fellows," (Petersdorf, 1978) and a chairman of medicine in this study complained about the Balkanization of internal medicine. Along with subspecialization, notice was taken of "more science in the specialty" and "getting M.D.s with cell and molecular biology training."

More important yet is the increasing differentiation caused by the split between clinical research and basic research. One chairman had said, "If you look at the research going on in the departments, it's being done by Ph.D.s." And the sample showed basic scientists appointed throughout the clinical specialties. That trend was viewed with anything but universal acceptance. Among the reasons given by a dual-career couple for leaving their jobs was that "they thought Ph.D.s could do research as well as M.D.s." A junior faculty M.D.–Ph.D. in medicine said that he could have done as well without the Ph.D. training, and a distinguished professor of pediatrics, also an M.D.–Ph.D., stated that "we have the best genetics in man, we know the most about man" and stressed that the physician's understanding of man was extremely important to medical research. And there was little evidence of desire or action taking place to integrate the activities of basic scientists with clinical researchers in the department.

The research culture is also typified by the interdisciplinarity that results from a continuing refinement of specialization into subspecialization. And the medical school, like the arts and sciences college—but again in the forefront—was the site of much interdisciplinary activity: "Departments are not the best way to do research." The interdisciplinary nature of medical faculty jobs was evidenced by the common involvement in the recruiting process of faculty members outside the hiring departments.

So, the research culture is alive and well in academic medicine, linking the medical school with tight bonds to the greater university and exercising a strong influence on the faculty mobility environment. As Dr. Stossel (1987) said, "The entire medical establishment recognized the importance of science and accepted the leadership of scientifically trained physicians with track records in research."

THE REAL WORLD

The real world enters the medical school through the doors of the hospital, which is both a teaching site and a research base for the medical faculty. The hospital is the place where the medical academician works. It is a workplace that differs from the academic setting in its day-in, day-out, year-in, year-out service to patients (Ebert, 1977).

But apart from the indirect effects of environment, the hospital directly affects medical faculty mobility in more concrete ways. The hospital is frequently the provider of a significant portion of the space that was a recurring feature of recruitment in this study: The senior recruit who "met with several other heads in the hospital" but could not reach a final solution of the space problem and was still hoping for a "formula" was a common figure.

The hospital furnishes collective and individual income through the faculty practice plan ("50 percent of faculty salaries" in one department in the study). The hospital may also have a hire-and-fire role in a faculty career, especially in a school where tenure does not carry a salary commitment. In one such school in this sample, a pathologist with a full-time faculty appointment was "laid off," according to his former chairman, because the hospital could not afford to continue his salary. And the hospital makes contributions to medical education (employing residents, for example) and research (through equipment and staff support) that influence faculty decisions.

In this study, the hospital's influence was seen first at the outset of the mobility process, in the decision to recruit. The program growth that was the main reason for recruiting was frequently an extension of patient care, either directly or in clinical research, and sometimes the new position resulted from money allocated by the hospital. Hospital needs were stressed by chairs who had heavy clinical obligations and so were "always on the lookout for young people who are promising."

Hospitals and medical school departments conducted joint searches in some cases; in others, a hospital division that was "independent" searched for, selected, and then submitted the credentials for approval of a candidate for a faculty appointment. The appointment might be confirmed by a hospital director, and the new faculty member would not "get an appointment letter from the university for about a year."

In attracting senior people, the hospital was a useful recruiting tool. The advantages for a newly appointed professor were noted by the chairman who described the lure of a "very large clinical base in a preeminent hospital," and a new professor referred to having successfully negotiated "my own inpatient ward, my own unit with my own house staff."

More to the point were expressions of the real-world demands of the faculty job, from the pathology chairman who was "constantly worrying about billing and unhappy patients" because of his dependence on patient care income, to the anesthesia chairman who knew that the size of his faculty had to be sufficient to meet the need for "one anesthetist for every two operating rooms."

In spite of the stress of combining ivory tower and real world, I met no medical faculty members who suggested operating in any other way. The blend of academics and practice was part of the accepted landscape and, indeed, constituted the special attraction of academic medicine for many. As Dr. Stossel (1987) remarked about his vanished medical school, it was unique because it had "its cutting edge of service in the university."

AT THE INTERSECTION

Dr. Stossel's scientifically trained physicians and cutting edge of service meet in the medical school, and the meeting is reflected in this study of faculty perpetuation. In addition to the preceding observations about separate research and clinical influences, the study provides four major insights into the organizational environment, structure, and behavior of the medical school.

First, the study suggests that the labor market of the medical academic marketplace is constrained by a number of factors. Chief among them are the multiple career options of the participants in the market, with respect not only to practice setting (private, academic, etc.) that conceivably could be available at any time, but also specialty and subspecialty at the beginning of the medical career.

Chairs spoke of efforts to present their specialties in an attractive light to medical students—addressing "the sophomore class in the medical school" in an attempt to encourage the choice of specialty. This was a type of intervention that made good sense because several of the faculty members queried had selected a specialty for reasons reflecting the influence of an authority figure, such as the lecturer who "was extremely dynamic and simply made a superb presentation."

Chairs also saw the circumstances surrounding the choice of academic medicine as a market problem. Lack of tutorial (mentoring) programs was noted and the need "to find the very best first-year medical students and begin to cultivate them." Proposed remedies focused on the research experience, with plans of professional associations to "subsidize research nationally with a heavily endowed program for residents" and to create a training program with a "full year of research in the middle." The relationship to the research culture (the ivory tower) discussed earlier and to the preferences of physicians who choose academic medicine for teaching and research were evident.

In addition, chairs targeted the subspecialization noted as a part of the research culture as a problem in the market, especially connected with a lack of training opportunities. There were "not enough people coming through the academic training programs to satisfy some subspecialties" and "not enough trainee slots."

Second, the findings show organizational stability. Contrary to popular opinion both within the medical school and in the greater university, the medical faculty is not a highly mobile group. In the workforce of 4,311 faculty members represented in this study, there were appointments amounting to less than 5 percent of that figure and terminations of only 3 1/2 percent. In both cases, the proportions were favorable in comparison to those of my arts and sciences study, with appointments slightly higher and terminations considerably lower, as shown by the following data:

	Medical		Arts & Sciences	
	No.	%	No.	%
Total faculty	4,311	100.0	3,302	100.0
Appointments	207	4.8	137	4.1
Terminations	149	3.5	167	5.1

The new appointments covered by the study were reported a year later as largely successful, with both chairs and appointees expressing satisfaction. Chairs were quite specific in their positive comments about junior faculty members as being "very stable and a collaborative type of individual," having "tremendously good people management techniques," or adding "a new area of expertise." The majority of new appointees, as well, were satisfied with academic medicine and their jobs.

In the area of termination, there was a very low number of retirements—and most of the retirees had not really left, that is, they were still actively contributing to the work of the department. The majority of the faculty members who moved from one job to another had stayed in academic medicine; in fact, the loss to higher education from the medical faculty was essentially no greater in proportion than the loss from the arts and sciences, thus calling into question the widely held notion that a great many people leave academic medicine for private practice.

Tenure or reappointment denials were scarce in the sample, although several resignations may have been marginally voluntary. Even considering those situations, the mobility environment in the medical school was not a churning scene—a small percentage of the medical faculty was moving into or out of the organization.

Perhaps a negative effect on organizational stability occurred at another level: in the lack of congruence between the reports of chairs and departed faculty members, for example, or in the shifting goals reported in the case study in chapter 5. Where chairs and their former faculty members disagreed so widely in their remarks, one wonders about organizational health. And where a dean made a decision in a reactive vacuum, one laments the absence of strategic planning. The chairman who described long-range plans in medical schools as covering "a year or a year and a half" was describing a condition of organizational instability, where planning consisted of wish lists of things the chairs or division chiefs wanted and efforts to find the money for them.

Anecdotal information from the minority, too, suggested dissonance in the organization that might be more widespread than was revealed through the focus of this study. The faculty member who bemoaned the isolation from the rest of the university represented a yearning for a more academic environment; faculty members who had left complained of "frustrations with chairman" and "lack of support"—perceptions damaging to the organization. But, basically, the examination of faculty recruitment and termination revealed the medical school as a stable organization.

The study also touches on three factors that might be considered aspects of organizational differentiation: academic rank, tenure status, and professional orientation. The greatest mobility in the study occurred at the assistant professor rank (as could be expected, and as was also the case in the arts and sciences study). Recruiting procedures differed by rank as well: Junior faculty recruitment was conducted in a relatively informal manner and was often associated with program growth or expansion; searches for senior people were carefully executed and were more likely to result from replacement needs. The contrast might be summed up in the chairman's remark that "assistant professors don't meet deans" but that the dean was useful in senior recruitment.

On the other hand, tenure status was not a variable in the processes investigated in the study, although there was the implication of a difference in the job, with the faculty that was not tenure-eligible carrying a larger share of the clinical load and having less—but still some—protected time for research. Also having a minimal effect was the idea of local and cosmopolitan, which did not fit the medical faculty in the traditional way—that is, inhibiting or stimulating movement—but rather only in destination of movement as between academic medicine (cosmopolitan) and private practice (local).

Third, the study shows that the clinical science department of the medical school occupies a unique position in academia, affecting chairs in particular, but also faculty members at other levels in the department. The financial responsibility that exists at the departmental level imbues the clinical chair with a considerable degree of power. The chairs in this study were responsible for sizeable annual budgets ($12 million was a specific example), largely department-generated, and the consequent financial independence affected recruiting; the situation where the new faculty member's salary "comes out of clinical earnings" and the chair had "considerable autonomy" in deciding to recruit was not unusual.

At the beginning of the recruitment process, therefore, the clinical chair had the authority to proceed, so long as he or she could afford it. The control exercised by the chair was remarkable for an academic setting: "I decide what we need," "I make the decision," and "my personal vision drives the recruitment" were statements that represented the norm in the clinical sciences. Appointments were subject to academic constraints (the ivory tower's influence), but, as long as the real world of budget allowed, recruitment was subject to little other control. The search process was similarly controlled or directed by the chair; although the selection process was somewhat more democratic, the chairman who compared the decision-making process to "going into a harbor among buoys" was decidedly in the minority.

Add to these aspects of organizational behavior the longevity of a clinical chairmanship—averaging eleven years and ranging up to twenty-seven years in this sample—and we saw a very strong role delineated. The person in this role, thus, developed his or her own management strategies that included soliciting financially lucrative industry partnerships, establishing departmental fund-raising functions, and spinning off business operations separate from the academic and clinical mission.

Power similar to that enjoyed by the chair devolved to senior members of the faculty in positions such as division chief and program director and was especially evident in the conditions that senior faculty members placed on taking their new job. Those physicians were going to run their own show and "didn't want any interference." The organization acquiesced: "They gave him the world." Authority followed financial responsibility at other levels as well; junior faculty members might be hired by senior faculty members who were providing support until they obtained their own grant funds.

At all ranks and levels of responsibility, the new faculty member was expected to generate all or part of his or her own salary through research grants, patient care income, or both. The percentage differed by institution, but at only one of the schools in this sample was the contribution as low as 25 percent. (It was enlightening to me that the 25-percent institution was called a "hard money school," that is, salaries paid out of university funds rather than departmental income, by a new faculty member who had moved from another institution in the sample that required a larger percentage, which he characterized as a "soft money school"—obviously in relative rather than absolute terms.) Start-up funds might be available, but support would diminish as the faculty member established a research program—"We prime the pump, but we expect him to pick up 50 percent of his salary in grants." And the self-supporting nature of the medical faculty job was also a factor in terminations, where reappointment was denied because a department could not afford to keep someone who was not generating grant support.

Fourth, the study indicates a closed system of faculty recruiting—particularism as opposed to universalism. The latter would entail broad communication of information about an opening, consideration of a variety of applicants, and careful (and reasonably objective) procedures applied to selection in a participatory process. Particularism, on the other hand, denotes a recruitment and selection process that is limited in scope and heavily dependent on subjectivity.

Recruitment of professionals is usually a particularistic process. The degree of autonomy accorded a professional makes "fitting in" a requirement in order to ensure support for the values of the organization, and the attribute of fit is thought to be best determined within a known circle of contacts—witness the chief of cardiology who recruited within his "universe"—and by subjective evaluation. Particularism in recruitment reduces the degree of uncertainty in a professional appointment.

In this study, although faculty positions were advertised (a universalistic practice) in many cases, the advertising was clearly neither effective nor expected to be effective. Chairs considered advertising mainly an affirmative action requirement; a chairman's assertion that advertising was not "the most effective or efficient" recruiting method was typical. Newly appointed faculty members also discounted the method, often mentioning that they had seen an ad but had not considered the position until contacted personally.

Consequently, the process shifted immediately to one of particularism—"the real way we do it is to start calling people who train good fellows." And beyond that kind of approach was the more mutual endeavor, found in the speculative applications of junior faculty members and the use of contacts at the senior level where, for example, the successful candidate "happened to know the people on the committee."

Applicant pools were small; indeed, there was a preponderance of single-candidate recruitments, some related to recruitments of senior faculty members who had brought staff with them, but many the targeting of a specific person via the sponsorship of a colleague. A model of particularism was present in the case study at the end of chapter 5, in which the division chief and three junior faculty members all were personally recruited (as were the four faculty members who moved to other jobs).

A broader model of particularism is the internal labor market in academic medicine. In this sample, where there was a large proportion of appointments of house staff to faculty positions, the actual observation of the resident or fellow permitted a depth of evaluation that was reassuring to the department, summed up by the chairman who commented that an assistant professor had been appointed because of "qualities that I—and all of the other department members—had observed when he was here as a resident." Indeed, the internal labor market of the medical school may be the primary example of a closed recruitment system in today's universe of organizations.

CONCLUSION

The academic physician's world is a mixture of the academic and the practical; indeed, the medical school is a model of applied science. Physicians are recruited to academic medicine in a tight market where other opportunities abound and where choice of specialty and subspecialty may occur in a relatively short period of time, during which it becomes necessary to accelerate the socialization process. On the other hand, physicians who choose academic medicine tend to stick with it, suggesting a personality type that might be identified and nurtured.

Although the academic nature of the medical school is pronounced and pervasive, not all of the university's customs and mores have been accepted. Tenure status, for example, does not represent the division in a medical school that is present in the class structure of an arts and sciences college. Also, the clinical department is a miniature professional school itself, and the chair is a mini-dean, carrying responsibility and exercising authority in substance and manner different from that found in chairs elsewhere in the university.

In an intensification rather than total departure from standard operating procedure in the university, the medical school uses a closed system of recruiting much more extensively. Particularism is reflected in the almost exclusive use of personal contacts for single-candidate recruitments, but the extreme application of the principle is found in the heavy incidence of appointment of a school's own residents and fellows to the faculty. Particularism thus narrows the risk inherent in hiring professionals; the extreme to which it is carried in the medical school may also hamper innovation and creativity within a faculty.

So much for the present. And what of the future? A primary consideration would be the labor market for academic physicians: Will it change and if so, how? The study alludes to several factors that will influence the supply and demand of medical academicians in the years ahead. First, the expansion of academic medicine responsible for much of the recruiting activity in the study is unlikely to continue; there will be far fewer faculty positions created by new programs and expansion of existing programs. Second, the government regulation and control of income in private practice noted by respondents may turn the medical student's thoughts toward academic medicine at an earlier stage in the career decision-making process (and may in fact populate medical schools with a somewhat differently motivated faculty). Third, although the subspecialist is the rule, the generalist is often the need, especially as patient care continues to be an important source of income for the medical school. These probabilities—less or no growth, a higher profile for academic medicine, and de-emphasis of subspecialization—suggest that the market for academic physicians will ease over a period of years.

A second consideration lies in the changes that are taking place in higher education today, especially in terms of public accountability. The legitimacy of the goals of the research university (the type of institution to which medical schools are attached) is being questioned by the American public. In a similar vein, the medical school—or, more accurately, the academic medical center—is undergoing public scrutiny. In addition, as the information society of a postindustrial economy has spawned a number of organizations similar to universities, so has there been a proliferation of organizations similar in whole or in part to academic medical centers. Consequently, neither higher education in general nor medical schools in particular have retained a unique claim on certain resources. The search for new sources of financial support is leading to a greater reliance on business and industry; the activity that will take place in the new research buildings that are springing up on every medical campus may ultimately be administered through interesting new forms of alliance. And, of course, for the medical school the uncertain future of the structure and content of the American health care delivery system poses questions for the future. These intrusions of the external environment may have effects, both quantitative and qualitative, on medical faculty mobility.

A third, and highly important, consideration is the large question of the character of the medical school. Dr. Stossel portrayed a gloomy future, where the clinical investigator had disappeared and, as a result, the distinctive nature of the medical school had dissolved. It seems clear that the medical school's niche in higher education is dependent on its unique blend of ivory tower and real world, and that movement away from clinical investigation is in effect a regression to what Dr. Stossel called the "one-dimensionality of earlier times." The "two-platoon system" of basic and clinical research that appears to be developing in the medical school constitutes a future threat to the faculty member's notion of the practice of academic medicine that provided much of the rationale for actions taken by participants in this study.

Given future possibilities, illuminated by the research represented in this book, I am hazarding a few recommendations with respect to faculty perpetuation in the ever-changing environment of the medical school.

1. *Strategic planning is a critical need*. I do not mean the usual five-year plan that is a budgeting crutch, but rather a careful examination of institutional strengths and weaknesses, an assessment of environmental factors, and an appraisal of the degree of congruence in organizational and individual objectives. One of my respondents mentioned the need to identify "steeples of excellence" in the face of the knowledge that a medical school could not be everything to everyone; however, even at his school, there was no evidence that such a process was under way. Staffing has not been a well-planned feature of the medical school organization, but the greater constraints of the future will require attention to planning the size and scope of the faculty.

2. *Management concepts need revision*. Authoritarianism is a style that has been proved inadequate to the successful management of professionals. Among systems in place or those being introduced into some medical schools are provisions for chair review and maximum terms of service for chairs—measures that will serve to curb authoritarianism. I would suggest going a giant step further, to centralize income and broaden the base for faculty salaries to a school-wide rather than a departmental level, thus converting departmental autonomy to traditional

academic concerns of collegiality and peer review. Such a change in organizational culture could be beneficial at several points in the faculty mobility process.

3. *The clinical base of medical research must be preserved.* It is absolutely necessary for the medical school of the future to find ways for basic scientists to interact with their physician colleagues in the clinical departments. Alexander Pope, in a slightly different context, wrote that the proper study of mankind was man; certainly, the academic physicians of this study believed that to be true. But in present conditions, basic scientists are not sufficiently integrated into the clinical work of the department, a reality that is likely to deepen a division that was already being noticed by many of my respondents and that could easily affect the attraction of academic medicine for many potential faculty members.

A faculty member at one of the schools I visited remarked in conversation that academic medicine was something of an oxymoron. And indeed, we have seen that physicians play a role in the academic marketplace that is unique because of the inherent contradiction of terms in their chosen profession. Nevertheless, this study of faculty mobility, following the dictum that understanding the process by which a faculty maintains its immortality is central to the understanding of the institution, has revealed the strong academic foundation of the medical school. I trust that in a way this will serve to enhance and progress intraorganizational relationships in the university and its medical school.

Appendix A

Methodology

My study was exploratory, intended to result in a description of medical faculty mobility processes; I needed optimum information yield, of the sort available only through interviewing the people who could furnish the information. Consequently, I chose a simple qualitative methodology—a structured interview, content analysis, and descriptive statistics.[1] (I was guided in this choice by a desire to make this study similar to my earlier study of arts and sciences faculty,[2] so that data might be compared across studies.)

The first task of research design was to define the objective of the study, which resulted in the following statement:

Study Objective

To analyze the faculty recruitment and termination process in medical schools, in an organizational context.

Then, the conduct of the research might be illustrated by a progression of units following from the study objective (see figure).

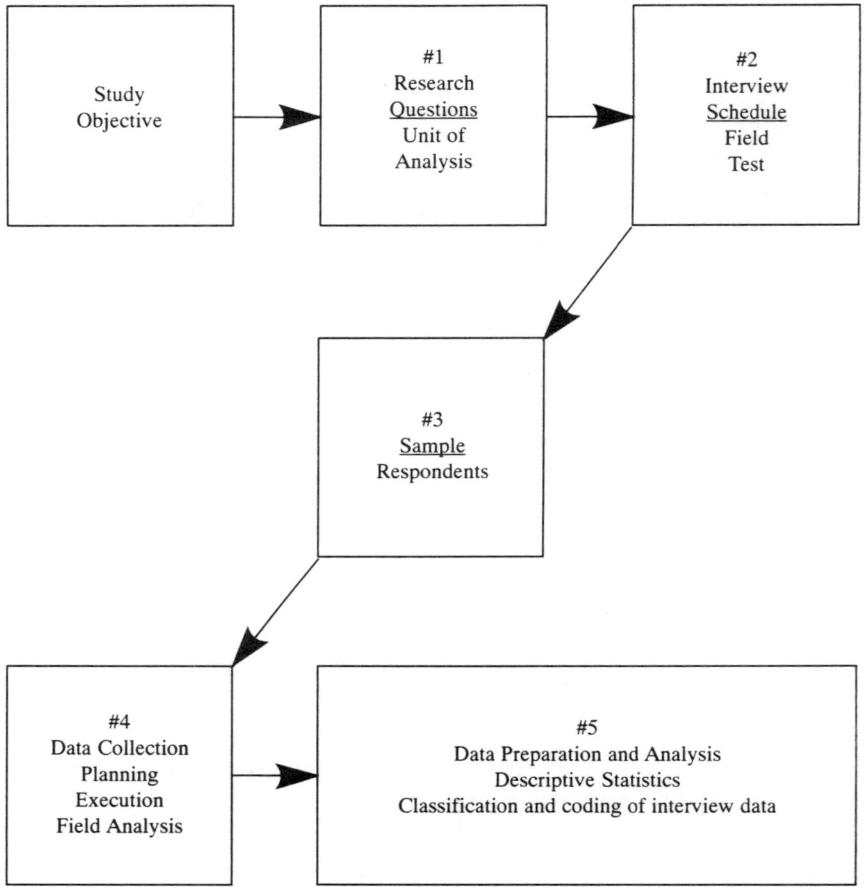

RESEARCH QUESTIONS/UNIT OF ANALYSIS

Research questions are important both for what they are and for what they are not. The great advantage of qualitative over quantitative research is the richness of human experience that can be captured in personal encounters with respondents. Therefore, it is necessary to be guided by broad questions that do not restrict the investigation. On the other hand, the great disadvantage of qualitative research is the seemingly limitless possibilities that could impede adequate analysis and description. Research questions should provide a framework for inquiry that will prevent tangential interludes and unfocused observations.

Trying to strike a balance, I framed the following basic research questions for the study:

1. What are the existing practices and criteria for discovering and evaluating medical faculty candidates?
2. How are selection decisions made?
3. What are the circumstances of medical faculty terminations?
4. What is the effect of market characteristics on the organization through its personnel processes?
5. What is the effect of institutional policies on the organization through its personnel processes?

Each of these questions can be subdivided into indicators of specificity; for example, with respect to question 3: What is the incidence of denial of tenure for assistant professors? What degree of mobility exists for associate and full professors? When medical faculty members move voluntarily, why do they do it and where do they go?

Another essential ingredient in the balance of the study is the unit of analysis, which plays an important role in tying the study results to the study objective, as well as furnishing additional definition to the research task. The unit of analysis should focus the research questions to deepen understanding of the process. It would appear that a general approach—such as asking administrators to enumerate procedures—would not reach the heart of the process. Rather, it would be preferable to examine an actual personnel action, asking questions about specific incidents, and then using the data so obtained to identify patterns in the process.

Therefore, the unit of analysis for this study was an actual appointment or termination of a medical faculty member, bounded to provide a specific set of actions for comparative purposes,[3] as follows:

- Full-time appointments occurring in the 1987–1988 academic year.
- Full-time terminations occurring in the 1986–1987 academic year.

("Full-time" in this study means a paid position for which all income is derived from a university source, and because joint appointments in more than one department are common in medicine, the position is that of the primary appointment.)

INTERVIEW GUIDE/FIELD TEST

With decisions made about the research questions and the unit of analysis, the next step was the development of an instrument that would enable me to analyze the personnel actions, answer the questions, and reach my study objective. I wanted to ask open-ended questions during the interview that would elicit information about those faculty members who left, whether voluntarily or involuntarily, and those who joined the organization. I also wanted to ask questions about the circumstances of the appointment or termination. I was fortunate in this instance in having an interview guide that had worked well in my previous study, and so I made a few modifications to fit the medical environment and conducted a field test in order to make sure that the questions would flow well in the actual interview situation and produce the information I was seeking. I field-tested the interview guide in the Department of Medicine at Duke University Medical Center and made only minor adjustments to the instrument as a result.[4]

SAMPLE/RESPONDENTS

Unlike many quantitative studies, where randomization is an important element, the typical qualitative study relies on a sample that is tailored to the research. In this instance, again for reasons of comparability, I chose to study the medical schools that were counterparts of the arts and sciences colleges of research universities that were the setting for my previous study. Three of the schools were separate institutions within state systems, and three were professional schools of private research universities. All were in urban locations; one shared a campus with the undergraduate college and nonmedical professional schools. As to geographic location, two were in the East, two were in the Midwest, one was in the West, and one was in the Southwest. The six schools employed 4,624 of the 44,621 full-time faculty members in the clinical sciences in 1988 (these numbers are not limited to M.D.s but include all faculty members in the clinical sciences regardless of degree type).

The prestige and emphases of the schools varied. In a reputational ranking of ninety-four medical schools, three of the schools in this study ranked in the top fifteen and three were in the category from twenty to fifty.[5] In terms of emphasis, three of the schools were judged well above average in both undergraduate and graduate medical education, research emphasis, and research funding (these were also the schools ranked in the top fifteen); one was above average in research emphasis but average in the other factors; one was below average on all factors; and one, predominantly oriented toward undergraduate medical education, was also slightly above average in research emphasis but slightly below average in graduate medical education and research funding.[6]

The study included all clinical specialties. Where a subspecialty was found as a separate department in only one school in the sample, it was merged into the specialty in which it was contained in the other five schools (e.g., neurosurgery was included in surgery). The study also included pathology, which might be considered a basic science. (At one school, I asked the chairman of pathology whether he considered his specialty a basic or clinical science and he said, "yes.") Generally, I followed the rule of including in the study all departments categorized as medical, surgical, behavioral, and hospital-based,[7] the last group including pathology. For purposes of this study, the categorization of specialties is as follows:

Medical:	Dermatology, family medicine, internal medicine, neurology, and pediatrics.
Surgical:	Obstetrics and gynecology, ophthalmology, orthopedic surgery, otolaryngology, and surgery.
Behavioral:	Psychiatry.
Hospital-based:	Anesthesia, pathology, and radiology.

I did not include basic sciences in the study for three reasons: I was concerned primarily with the physician (M.D.) in the medical school; faculty personnel practices and markets in the basic science departments are more clearly aligned with those of the natural sciences of the arts and sciences college; and the low incidence of personnel activity in basic science departments during the period studied would have prevented adequate representation.

Choosing the respondents was not a difficult task. I decided to follow the successful model of the arts and sciences study in talking to the chair of each department where appointments or terminations had occurred about those actions, and to new appointees about their own appointments. A departure from the earlier study, made possible by the national records available on the whereabouts of physicians,[8] was a mailed questionnaire, with open-ended questions adapted from the interview guide, to faculty members who had left their positions. (A few of these physicians turned up as appointments elsewhere and were personally interviewed, and some were interviewed by phone, either initially owing to proximity or as a clarifying follow-up to the returned questionnaire.)

I enjoyed a high success rate in completed interviews, which included all of the appropriate chairs (or in three cases, knowledgeable senior designees); I also interviewed division chiefs in some large departments. Of the 207 new appointments, I was able to interview 168 of the newly appointed faculty members; out of the 131 terminations (excluding retirements and deaths), I was able to locate and send questionnaires or otherwise contact 104 faculty members, with 52 completions. In all, my respondents (including chairs and division chiefs) totaled 300, including 103 full professors, 35 associate professors, 150 assistant professors, and 12 instructors or associates (not house staff) in 70 departments. Medical schools make heavy use of nontenure-track positions; therefore, the respondent group of 300 included 83 persons with nontenurable positions: 10 full professors, 17 associate professors, 50 assistant professors, and 6 instructors or associates.[9]

DATA COLLECTION

Data collection may be considered in three parts: planning, execution, and field analysis. Planning consists generally of obtaining any preliminary materials, deciding what has to be done on site, and making advance arrangements. Execution is the data collection, the interviewing itself. Analysis of data while in the field is a mechanism for developing a familiarity with the site data prior to the full analysis that comes later (and it's fun).[10]

Planning

Initially, the Chancellor for Health Affairs at my institution wrote a letter to the top administrator at each of the schools I hoped to include in the study, describing the study and asking for a contact person on campus. Fortunately, everyone contacted agreed to participate. I then obtained a list of appointments and terminations for the appropriate periods, as well as school bulletins and written procedures governing appointment and termination. The list of appointments and terminations included department, rank, tenure status, and in the case of terminations, type (dismissal, voluntary resignation, retirement, or death). For each school, I prepared a tentative summary of the initial data; I say tentative because, as in the case of the arts and sciences study, no school's list was entirely accurate and field modifications were necessary.

One school refused to provide information about terminated faculty members, a stance that necessitated my spending several hours in the school's library comparing school bulletins from year to year to compile my own list, subsequently checked with department chairs as I talked with them.

Execution

Upon arrival on campus, I arranged interview appointments by telephone (and once again learned the value of friendly and competent secretaries and assistants). Generally, regardless of the degree of warmth in the official greeting (which ranged from high at two schools to nil at one), once I had negotiated some kind of work space and message-taking and got on with it, I was well received.[11] Several of the faculty members with whom I talked were enthusiastic about my research, and almost all were interested. Only one faculty member explicitly refused to be interviewed—an assistant professor of family medicine who considered my project an invasion of privacy.

I conducted all personal interviews in the faculty member's office or laboratory in as unobtrusive a manner as could be accomplished. I recorded responses verbatim on the previously prepared interview form (using shorthand), dictating the interviews at the end of the day for transcription later.

Field Analysis

Field analysis was quite helpful in giving me a holistic sense of the campus results as I was collecting the data. For example, a spreadsheet comparison of chairman and appointee responses on selected questions—their respective interviews might be days apart—was a good check on my perceptions. Another useful exercise was keeping a list of persons I was not able to interview, noting characteristics, in order to maintain appropriate representation (for example, if I was unable to maximize interviews in radiology at one school, I would be especially careful to get a better response in radiology departments at the others). I summarized the data and wrote a site memo at the end of each site visit. Consequently, at the end of each visit, I had developed a familiarity with and a comprehensive view of the faculty personnel activity at that medical school, as well as some experience in handling the data.

DATA PREPARATION AND ANALYSIS

At the conclusion of the field research, I had two data components to be prepared for analysis: descriptive statistics and interview data. The descriptive statistics consisted of the numbers collected—appointments, involuntary terminations, voluntary resignations, retirements, and deaths—to be placed within parameters of institution, rank, specialty, type of appointment, etc. The descriptive statistics provided a framework for the study, telling me the "where" and "what" of the activity.

I checked the interview data twice, once in the field at the time of dictation and again when I compared transcribed drafts of the interviews with original notes. I cut copies of the final interview forms into sections corresponding to the research questions and pasted the sections onto color-coded (by school) index cards. I then assigned categorical coding to all of the index cards, providing each with an eight-character code designating school, specialty, and role of interviewee (for example, XYZPSY1C, which meant school, psychiatry, the first subject in an interview with a chairman); a four-character code establishing type of action (appointment or termination), with a fifth character for type of termination; and a four-character code for academic rank, with a fifth character for tenure status. All of the coding I used was non-numerical and relatively self-explanatory.[12] This initial coding permitted aggregation of the interview data for analysis in various ways. I also coded themes within the interview data where I had noted certain repetitions during data collection (for example, references to spouse employment); additional codes emerged from further familiarity with the responses as I worked with the data.[13] I used content analysis concomitantly with the "fine-coding" task to develop classifications, such as negative or positive response, and to furnish discrete quantifiable items, as well as to assess the meanings that were being conveyed by the faculty respondents.[14] In preparing the data chapters, two through five, I maintained a list of verbatim quotes used, classified by institution type, medical specialty, academic rank, and sex, in order to ensure adherence to the composition of the personnel activity studied.

The ultimate data analysis occurred in the writing itself. As I wrote, I tried to keep in mind Mintzberg's seven basic adjectives for what he called "direct" research: descriptive, simple ("inelegant" methodologies), inductive, systematic, real, supported (by anecdotal data), and integrative (creating synthesis).[15] The result, I believe, is a book that takes a direct approach to the investigation of medical faculty mobility.

NOTES

1. John Van Maanen suggested in the introduction to *Varieties of Qualitative Research* (Beverly Hills: Sage, 1982) that the organizational researcher carries certain axiomatic-like beliefs or principles, including analytic induction, proximity, and descriptive focus. Analytic induction proceeds from a primary data base of the specific and local within which patterns may or may not be found; proximity depends on first-hand accounts; and descriptive focus has to do with ontological inquiry—a description of what is occurring in a given place or time—where the aims of revelation and disclosure take precedence over explanation and prediction (p. 16).

2. Dolores L. Burke, *A New Academic Marketplace* (Westport, Conn.: Greenwood Press, 1988).

3. Robert K. Yin pointed out the importance of the unit of analysis in focusing the research questions and also the need for specific time boundaries (*Case Study Research: Design and Methods*, Beverly Hills: Sage, 1984).

4. The use of a structured interview, as well as the selection of respondents directly connected to the unit of analysis, increases the reliability of the research. The validity of the research is assured through the interview content and the sample (respondents and institutions). See, for example, discussions of reliability and validity in qualitative research in Paul Diesing, *Patterns of Discovery in the Social Sciences* (Chicago: Aldine, 1971), and Margaret D. LeCompte and Judith Preissle Goetz, "Problems of Reliability and Validity in Ethnographic Research," *Review of Educational Research* 52 (1982): 31–60. The multisite nature of the sample strengthens the generalizability of the study, although this qualitative inductive research lends itself better to analytical generalization than to the statistical generalization associated with sampling techniques. For discussion of the differences between quantitative and qualitative research in this regard, see Robert K. Yin, *Case Study Research: Design and Methods* (Beverly Hills: Sage, 1984), and Robert E. Herriott and William A. Firestone, "Multisite Qualitative Policy Research: Optimizing Description and Generalizability," *Educational Researcher* 12 (1983): 14–19.

5. Jonathan R. Cole and James A. Lipton, "The Reputations of American Medical Schools," *Social Forces* 55 (1977): 662–684.

6. Michael B. McShane and Charles R. Sherman, *Exploratory Analysis of Medical School Characteristics and Empirical Classifications of Medical Schools* (Washington: Association of American Medical Colleges, 1977).

7. These categories are taken from a National Research Council report, *On the Status of Medical School Faculty and Clinical Research Manpower 1968–1990*.

8. The sources I used were *ABMS Compendium of Certified Medical Specialists 1988–89* (Evanston, Ill.: American Board of Medical Specialists, 1988) and the AMA Physician Profile data base, the latter searched for me by the staff of the Division of Survey and Data Resources of the American Medical Association, Chicago, Illinois.

9. See note 4 above.

10. For the recognition that such field devices as writing memos are fun, and that it is important to protect time to have fun in projects, I am indebted to Matthew B. Miles and A. Michael Huberman in *Qualitative Data Analysis: A Sourcebook of New Methods* (Beverly Hills: Sage, 1984).

11. Theodore Caplow has noted that being interviewed is an inherently satisfying experience, perhaps because of interaction. "Somewhere in the course of socialization, interaction comes to be as 'natural,' as spontaneous, and as essential to the maintenance of the psyche as is the continuation of metabolism to the maintenance of the organism." Caplow also pointed out that the interview benefits from the system of expectations developed in it—it is a departure from conversations that have been threatening, frustrating, confusing, boring—and is, therefore, satisfying to the respondent. ("The Dynamics of Information Interviewing," *American Journal of Sociology* 62 (1956): 65–171.)

12. Here I followed the advice of Miles and Huberman that although words (and letters) may be more unwieldy than numbers, they enable "thick description."

13. The data reduction (preliminary analysis) of coding and categorizing has been said to generate a common language of concepts to guide further data analysis. (Matthew B. Miles, "Qualitative Data as an Attractive Nuisance: The Problems of Analysis," *Administrative Science Quarterly* 24 (1979): 590–601.)

14. Martin Bulmer pointed out that conceptual guidance in empirical studies comes from such facets as the logical analysis of a process, working back from regularities in the research data, and the respondents' own concepts, definitions, and experience. ("Concepts in the Analysis of Qualitative Data," *Sociological Review* 27 (1979): 651–677.)

15. Henry Mintzberg, "An Emerging Strategy of 'Direct' Research," *Administrative Science Quarterly* 24 (1979): 582–589.

Appendix B

Study Data

The following schedules provide detailed summaries of the data collected for this study from the six medical schools visited.

Appointments. All full-time faculty appointments reported for the academic year 1987–1988, listed by school and academic rank within categories of specialty and status (tenure track or not tenure track).

Terminations. All terminations, whether by voluntary resignation, dismissal, retirement, or death, reported for the academic year 1986–1987, listed by school and academic rank within categories of specialty and status.

Respondents. All respondents in the study, listed by school and academic rank within categories of specialty and status.

Size of departments. Total population represented by sample in fall 1988, listed by school and academic rank within specialty.

Appointments.

Specialty and Status	Public School A				Private School B				Public School C				Private School D			
	Inst	Asst	Assc	Prof	Inst	Asst	Assc	Prof	Inst	Asst	Assc	Prof	Inst	Asst	Assc	Prof
ANESTHESIA																
Tenure Track						3										
Not Ten Track		4														
FAMILY MED																
Tenure Track										1					1	
Not Ten Track			1													
MEDICINE																
Tenure Track						10		1				1	1		1	
Not Ten Track		4					2			3			3			1
NEUROLOGY																
Tenure Track						4										
Not Ten Track		1														
NEUROSURGERY																
Tenure Track																
Not Ten Track		1														
OB-GYN																
Tenure Track					1	2				2				1		
Not Ten Track		4						1	1	1						
OPHTHALMOLOGY																
Tenure Track												1				
Not Ten Track																
ORTHOPED SURG																
Tenure Track																
Not Ten Track										1						
OTOLARYNGOLOGY																
Tenure Track			1							1						
Not Ten Track																
PATH/ LAB MED																
Tenure Track						1							1			
Not Ten Track	1									1						
PEDIATRICS																
Tenure Track						3	2			2		1		1		1
Not Ten Track							2	1		3						1
PSYCHIATRY																
Tenure Track						4				1						
Not Ten Track										1						
RADIOLOGY																
Tenure Track						14					1	1				
Not Ten Track		4		1										1		
RAD ONCOLOGY																
Tenure Track																
Not Ten Track																
PHYS/REHAB MED																
Tenure Track																
Not Ten Track													1			
SURGERY																
Tenure Track						4		1		5				2		
Not Ten Track		3								1						
UROLOGY																
Tenure Track																
Not Ten Track	1															
TOTAL																
Tenure Track	0	0	1	0	1	45	2	2	0	12	1	4	3	4	2	1
Not Ten Track	2	21	1	1	0	0	4	2	1	11	0	0	3	1	0	2
All	2	21	2	1	1	45	6	4	1	23	1	4	6	5	2	3

Private School E				Public School F				Specialty	Total				
Inst	Asst	Assc	Prof	Inst	Asst	Assc	Prof	and Status	Inst	Asst	Assc	Prof	All
								ANESTHESIA					
	1		1					Tenure Track	0	4	0	1	5
				2	1	1		Not Ten Track	2	5	1	0	8
								FAMILY MED					
								Tenure Track	0	1	1	0	2
					1			Not Ten Track	0	1	1	0	2
								MEDICINE					
	7				1			Tenure Track	1	18	1	2	22
				1	2			Not Ten Track	4	9	2	1	16
								NEUROLOGY					
	1							Tenure Track	0	5	0	0	5
								Not Ten Track	0	1	0	0	1
								NEUROSURGERY					
								Tenure Track	0	0	0	0	0
								Not Ten Track	0	1	0	0	1
								OB-GYN					
	9							Tenure Track	1	14	0	0	15
		1			1			Not Ten Track	1	6	1	1	9
								OPHTHALMOLOGY					
								Tenure Track	0	0	0	1	1
								Not Ten Track	0	0	0	0	0
								ORTHOPED SURG					
	1							Tenure Track	0	1	0	0	1
								Not Ten Track	0	1	0	0	1
								OTOLARYNGOLOGY					
								Tenure Track	0	1	1	0	2
								Not Ten Track	0	0	0	0	0
								PATH/LAB MED					
	2							Tenure Track	1	3	0	0	4
			2					Not Ten Track	1	1	0	2	4
								PEDIATRICS					
	5	1	2		1			Tenure Track	0	12	3	4	19
			1		2	1	1	Not Ten Track	0	5	3	4	12
								PSYCHIATRY					
	3							Tenure Track	0	8	0	0	8
	2	2		1	3			Not Ten Track	1	6	2	0	9
								RADIOLOGY					
	4							Tenure Track	0	18	1	1	20
		1	1		2			Not Ten Track	0	7	1	2	10
								RAD ONCOLOGY					
	2							Tenure Track	0	2	0	0	2
								Not Ten Track	0	0	0	0	0
								PHYS/REHAB MED					
								Tenure Track	1	0	0	0	1
								Not Ten Track	0	0	0	0	0
								SURGERY					
	3	1	1					Tenure Track	0	14	1	2	17
			1		3		1	Not Ten Track	0	7	0	2	9
								UROLOGY					
								Tenure Track	0	0	0	0	0
								Not Ten Track	1	0	0	0	1
								TOTAL					
0	38	2	4	0	2	0	0	Tenure Track	4	101	8	11	124
0	2	4	5	4	15	2	2	Not Ten Track	10	50	11	12	83
0	40	6	9	4	17	2	2	All	14	151	19	23	207

Terminations.

Specialty	Public School A				Private School B				Public School C				Private School D			
and Status	Inst	Asst	Assc	Prof	Inst	Asst	Assc	Prof	Inst	Asst	Assc	Prof	Inst	Asst	Assc	Prof
ANESTHESIA																
Tenure Track										2	1				1	
Not Ten Track																
DERMATOLOGY																
Tenure Track																1
Not Ten Track																
FAMILY MED																
Tenure Track											1					
Not Ten Track																
MEDICINE																
Tenure Track						5	2	2			2	2				1
Not Ten Track		4		1												
NEUROLOGY																
Tenure Track						3										
Not Ten Track																
OB-GYN																
Tenure Track						2		1		1						1
Not Ten Track													1			
OPHTHALMOLOGY																
Tenure Track						1				1						
Not Ten Track																
OTOLARYNGOLOGY																
Tenure Track										1	1					
Not Ten Track																
PATH/ LAB MED																
Tenure Track						2		1			1					1
Not Ten Track		1								1						
PEDIATRICS																
Tenure Track						3				1	1			2	1	
Not Ten Track			1													
PSYCHIATRY																
Tenure Track				1		8				5					1	
Not Ten Track		2	1												1	
RADIOLOGY																
Tenure Track						3				1						
Not Ten Track																
PHYS/REHAB MED																
Tenure Track													1			
Not Ten Track													1			
SURGERY																
Tenure Track				1						1	2	1				
Not Ten Track			1							2						
TOTAL																
Tenure Track	0	0	0	2	0	27	2	4	0	13	9	3	1	2	3	4
Not Ten Track	0	7	3	1	0	0	0	0	0	3	0	0	2	0	1	0
All	0	7	3	3	0	27	2	4	0	16	9	3	3	2	4	4

Private School E				Public School F				Specialty	Total				
Inst	Asst	Assc	Prof	Inst	Asst	Assc	Prof	and Status	Inst	Asst	Assc	Prof	All
								ANESTHESIA					
	2	1	1					Tenure Track	0	4	3	1	8
				1	1			Not Ten Track	1	1	0	0	2
								DERMATOLOGY					
			1		1	1		Tenure Track	0	1	1	2	4
								Not Ten Track	0	0	0	0	0
								FAMILY MED					
								Tenure Track	0	0	1	0	1
					1	1		Not Ten Track	0	1	1	0	2
								MEDICINE					
	2	1	4		3	1		Tenure Track	0	10	6	9	25
	4							Not Ten Track	0	8	0	1	9
								NEUROLOGY					
			1					Tenure Track	0	3	0	1	4
								Not Ten Track	0	0	0	0	0
								OB-GYN					
	5		1					Tenure Track	0	8	0	3	11
	1							Not Ten Track	1	1	0	0	2
								OPHTHALMOLOGY					
								Tenure Track	0	2	0	0	2
	1							Not Ten Track	0	1	0	0	1
								OTOLARYNGOLOGY					
								Tenure Track	0	1	1	0	2
								Not Ten Track	0	0	0	0	0
								PATH/LAB MED					
	1	1						Tenure Track	0	3	2	2	7
	2	1						Not Ten Track	0	4	1	0	5
								PEDIATRICS					
	1							Tenure Track	0	7	2	0	9
	1	1			2			Not Ten Track	0	3	2	0	5
								PSYCHIATRY					
			2					Tenure Track	0	13	1	3	17
	1			1				Not Ten Track	1	3	2	0	6
								RADIOLOGY					
								Tenure Track	0	4	0	0	4
	1				2			Not Ten Track	0	3	0	0	3
								PHYS/REHAB MED					
								Tenure Track	1	0	0	0	1
								Not Ten Track	1	0	0	0	1
								SURGERY					
	1		4		1		1	Tenure Track	0	3	2	7	12
		2				1		Not Ten Track	0	2	4	0	6
								TOTAL					
0	12	3	14	0	5	2	1	Tenure Track	1	59	19	28	107
0	11	4	0	2	6	2	0	Not Ten Track	4	27	10	1	42
0	23	7	14	2	11	4	1	All	5	86	29	29	149

Respondents.

Specialty and Status	Public School A Inst	Asst	Assc	Prof	Private School B Inst	Asst	Assc	Prof	Public School C Inst	Asst	Assc	Prof	Private School D Inst	Asst	Assc	Pro
ANESTHESIA																
Tenure Track				1		2		2		1		1			1	1
Not Ten Track		4														
DERMATOLOGY																
Tenure Track																1
Not Ten Track																
FAMILY MED																
Tenure Track				1						1	1	2			1	1
Not Ten Track			1													
MEDICINE																
Tenure Track				1		7		3				2	3		1	3
Not Ten Track		6					2			2			1			
NEUROLOGY																
Tenure Track				1		3		1								
Not Ten Track		1														
NEUROSURGERY																
Tenure Track			1													
Not Ten Track																
OB-GYN																
Tenure Track				1	1	1		1		3		1		1		1
Not Ten Track		4						1	1	1						
OPHTHALMOLOGY																
Tenure Track								1				1				
Not Ten Track																
ORTHOPED SURG																
Tenure Track												1				
Not Ten Track																
OTOLARYNGOLOGY																
Tenure Track			1	1						2	1	1				
Not Ten Track																
PATH/ LAB MED																
Tenure Track				2				1				1	1			2
Not Ten Track	1									1						
PEDIATRICS																
Tenure Track				1		4	1	1		3		2		2	1	2
Not Ten Track							2			3						1
PSYCHIATRY																
Tenure Track				1		3		1		4		1			1	1
Not Ten Track																
RADIOLOGY																
Tenure Track				1		9		1			1	2		1		1
Not Ten Track		3		1												
RAD ONCOLOGY																
Tenure Track																
Not Ten Track																
PHYS/REHAB MED																
Tenure Track													1		1	1
Not Ten Track																1
SURGERY																
Tenure Track				2		3		1		6	1	2		2		1
Not Ten Track		2	1							1						
UROLOGY																
Tenure Track																
Not Ten Track	1	1														
TOTAL																
Tenure Track	0	0	2	13	1	32	1	13	0	20	4	17	5	6	6	15
Not Ten Track	2	21	2	1	0	0	4	1	1	8	0	0	1	0	0	2
All	2	21	4	14	1	32	5	14	1	28	4	17	6	6	6	17

Private School E Inst	Private School E Asst	Private School E Assc	Private School E Prof	Public School F Inst	Public School F Asst	Public School F Assc	Public School F Prof	Specialty and Status	Total Inst	Total Asst	Total Assc	Total Prof	Total All
								ANESTHESIA					
	1	1	2				1	Tenure Track	0	4	2	8	14
					3	1		Not Ten Track	0	7	1	0	8
								DERMATOLOGY					
			2				1	Tenure Track	0	0	0	4	4
								Not Ten Track	0	0	0	0	0
								FAMILY MED					
							1	Tenure Track	0	1	2	5	8
					1			Not Ten Track	0	1	1	0	2
								MEDICINE					
	9		3		2	2	3	Tenure Track	3	18	3	15	39
	1			1	2			Not Ten Track	2	11	2	0	15
								NEUROLOGY					
			2					Tenure Track	0	3	0	4	7
								Not Ten Track	0	1	0	0	1
								NEUROSURGERY					
								Tenture Track	0	0	1	0	1
								Not Ten Track	0	0	0	0	0
								OB-GYN					
	9		2				1	Tenure Track	1	14	0	7	22
	1	1			1			Not Ten Track	1	7	1	1	10
								OPHTHALMOLOGY					
			1					Tenure Track	0	0	0	3	3
								Not Ten Track	0	0	0	0	0
								ORTHOPED SURG					
	1		1					Tenure Track	0	1	0	2	3
								Not Ten Track	0	0	0	0	0
								OTOLARYNGOLOGY					
								Tenure Track	0	2	2	2	6
								Not Ten Track	0	0	0	0	0
								PATH/LAB MED					
	2		1					Tenure Track	1	2	0	7	10
		1	2					Not Ten Track	1	1	1	2	5
								PEDIATRICS					
	5	1	3		1		1	Tenure Track	0	15	3	10	28
	1	1	1		2	1	1	Not Ten Track	0	6	4	3	13
								PSYCHIATRY					
	3		1				2	Tenure Track	0	10	1	7	18
	2	2		1	2			Not Ten Track	1	4	2	0	7
								RADIOLOGY					
	3		1				1	Tenure Track	0	13	1	7	21
		1	1		2			Not Ten Track	0	5	1	2	8
								RAD ONCOLOGY					
	1		1					Tenure Track	0	1	0	1	2
								Not Ten Track	0	0	0	0	0
								PHYS/REHAB MED					
								Tenure Track	1	0	1	1	3
								Not Ten Track	0	0	0	1	1
								SURGERY					
	4	1	2		1		2	Tenure Track	0	16	2	10	28
		2			3	1	1	Not Ten Track	0	6	4	1	11
								UROLOGY					
								Tenure Track	0	0	0	0	0
								Not Ten Track	1	1	0	0	2
								TOTAL					
0	38	3	22	0	4	2	13	Tenure Track	6	100	18	93	217
0	5	8	4	2	16	3	2	Not Ten Track	6	50	17	10	83
0	43	11	26	2	20	5	15	All	12	150	35	103	300

Size of Departments.

Specialty	Public School A						Private School B					Public School C		
	Inst	Asst	Assc	Prof	Total	Inst	Asst	Assc	Prof	Total	Inst	Asst	Assc	Prof
ANESTHESIA		15	2	14	31		17	10	6	33	2	21	8	4
DERMATOLOGY														
FAMILY MED		13	11	33	57							4	3	2
MEDICINE	11	73	45	85	214		127	85	83	295	2	65	47	85
NEUROLOGY		12	4	13	29		34	26	12	72				
NEUROSURGERY		7	3	13	23									
OB-GYN		12	6	22	40		14	12	14	40	1	8	7	8
OPHTHALMOLOGY							5	4	6	15		7	1	4
ORTHOPED SURG											5	1	3	3
OTOLARYNGOLOGY		6	2	5	13							6	3	2
PATH/ LAB MED		19	12	40	71		33	11	21	65		11	14	19
PEDIATRICS		21	17	38	76		52	33	22	107	8	23	12	15
PHYS/REHAB MED														
PSYCHIATRY		21	17	30	68		42	40	30	112	1	49	15	18
RADIOLOGY		23	14	49	86		39	26	16	81	1	20	11	12
RAD ONCOLOGY														
SURGERY		13	9	17	39		45	52	32	129		18	13	14
UROLOGY		4	2	4	10									
TOTAL	11	239	144	363	757		408	299	242	949	20	233	137	186
AVERAGE					45					86				

	Private School D					Private School E					Public School F				
Total	Inst	Asst	Assc	Prof	Total	Inst	Asst	Assc	Prof	Total	Inst	Asst	Assc	Prof	Total
35	2	3	2	3	10		28	26	6	60		8	6	4	18
							7	1	6	14		6	3	1	10
9	5	3	3	5	16							12	4	3	19
199	111	43	38	35	227		82	43	36	161		77	26	55	158
							18	8	13	39					
24	39	11	5	8	63		24	11	11	46		18	15	15	48
12	17	5	3	4	29		18	7	7	32					
12	13	10	5	6	34		9	6	10	25					
11															
44							32	9	23	64					
58	39	27	11	21	98		47	41	30	118		39	15	17	71
	5	10	5	1	21										
83	103	25	22	13	163		20	19	16	55		35	8	7	50
44	21	21	8	6	56		17	21	24	62		30	12	9	51
							12	6	7	25					
45	12	25	11	15	63		11	20	22	53		36	12	22	70
576	367	183	113	117	780		325	218	211	754		261	101	133	495
36					52					50					35

Appendix C

Medical Specialties and Subspecialties

Following is a list of medical specialties and subspecialties, with the year that board certification became available in the specialty or subspecialty; subspecialties are indented under specialty. (Data compiled by American Board of Medical Specialties, Evanston, Illinois.)

Specialty	Year
Allergy and immunology	1971
Diagnostic laboratory immunology	1986
Anesthesiology	1937
Critical care medicine	1986
Colon and rectal surgery	1934
Dermatology	1932
Dermatopathology	1974
Dermatological immunology	1985
Emergency medicine	1979
Family practice	1969
Geriatric medicine	1988
Sports medicine	1988
Internal medicine	1936
Cardiovascular disease	1941

Critical care medicine	1987
Diagnostic laboratory immunology	1986
Endocrinology and metabolism	1972
Gastroenterology	1941
Geriatric medicine	1988
Hematology	1972
Infectious disease	1972
Medical oncology	1973
Nephrology	1972
Pulmonary disease	1941
Rheumatology	1972
Neurological surgery	1939
Nuclear medicine	1971
Nuclear radiology	1957
Radioisotopic radiology	1974
Obstetrics and gynecology	1930
Gynecologic oncology	1974
Maternal and fetal medicine	1974
Reproductive endocrinology	1974
Ophthalmology	1917
Orthopedic surgery	1934
Hand surgery	1989
Otolaryngology	1924
Pathology	1935
Blood banking	1973
Chemical pathology	1950
Cytopathology	1989
Dermatopathology	1974
Forensic pathology	1959
Hematology	1952
Immunopathology	1983
Medical microbiology	1949
Neuropathology	1947
Pediatric pathology	1990
Radioisotopic pathology	1974

Pediatrics	1933
Diagnostic Laboratory Immunology	1986
Pediatric cardiology	1961
Pediatric critical care medicine	1987
Pediatric endocrinology	1978
Pediatric gastroenterology	1990
Pediatric hematology-oncology	1974
Pediatric nephrology	1974
Pediatric pulmonology	1986
Neonatal-perinatal medicine	1975
Physical medicine and rehabilitation	1947
Plastic surgery	1937
Hand surgery	1990
Preventive medicine	1948
Psychiatry and neurology	1934
Child and adolescent psychiatry	1959
Radiology	1932
Nuclear radiology	1957
Surgery	1937
Hand surgery	1989
Pediatric surgery	1975
Surgical critical care	1986
General vascular surgery	1982
Thoracic surgery	1945
Urology	1934

Bibliography

Anderson, Philip W., and Thomas A. Larson. *Mobility Characteristics of U.S. Medical School Faculty*. Washington, D.C.: Association of American Medical Colleges, 1975a.

______. *A Preliminary Analysis of Differential Characteristics between High and Low Mobile Medical School Faculty*. Washington, D.C.: Association of American Medical Colleges, 1975b.

Batshaw, Mark L., Leslie P. Plotnick, Brent G. Petty, Patricia K. Woolf, and E. David Mellitts. "Academic Promotion at a Medical School." *New England Journal of Medicine*. 318 (24 March 1988): 741–747.

Beaty, Harry N., David Babbott, Elizabeth J. Higgins, Paul Jolly, and Gerald S. Levey. "Research Activities of Faculty in Academic Departments of Medicine." *Annals of Internal Medicine*. 104 (January 1986): 90–97.

Bosk, Charles L. *Forgive and Remember*. Chicago: University of Chicago Press, 1979.

Burke, Dolores L. *A New Academic Marketplace*. Westport, Conn.: Greenwood Press, 1988.

Caplow, Theodore, and Reece McGee. *The Academic Marketplace*. New York: Basic Books, 1958.

Carnegie Commission on Higher Education. *Higher Education and the Nation's Health*. New York: McGraw-Hill, 1970.

Clark, Burton R. *The Academic Life: Small Worlds, Different Worlds*. Princeton, N.J.: Carnegie, 1987.

______. "Organizational Adaptation to Professionals: College Teaching." In *Professionalization*, ed. Howard M. Vollmer and Donald L. Mills. Englewood Cliffs, N.J.: Prentice-Hall, 1966.

Cole, Jonathan R., and James A. Lipton. "The Reputations of American Medical Schools." *Social Forces*. 55 (March 1977): 662–684.

Commonwealth Fund. *Prescription for Change*. New York: Commonwealth Fund, 1985.

Crawford, Steven A., and Christian N. Ramsey. "Resident and Faculty Perceptions of Faculty Qualifications." *Family Medicine*. 16 (November–December 1984): 210–214.

Davis, Wayne K., and William N. Kelley. "Factors Influencing Decisions to Enter Careers in Clinical Investigation." *Journal of Medical Education*. 57 (April 1982): 275–281.

Dill, David D. "Research as a Scholarly Activity: Context and Culture." In *Measuring Faculty Research Performance, New Directions for Institutional Research*, No. 50, ed. John W. Creswell. San Francisco: Jossey-Bass, 1986.

Ebert, Robert H. "Medical Education in the United States." *Daedalus*. 106 (Winter 1977): 171–184.

Ellwein, Leon B., Mohamed Khachab, and Robert H. Waldman. "Assessing Research Productivity: Evaluating Journal Publication Across Academic Departments." *Academic Medicine*. 64 (June 1989): 319–325.

Flexner, Abraham. *Medical Education in the United States and Canada*. New York: The Carnegie Foundation for the Advancement of Teaching, 1910.

Friedman, Paul J. "Faculty Renewal: Modeling the Impact of the End of Mandatory Retirement in the University of California Medical Schools." *Academic Medicine*. 64 (July 1989): 372–377.

Funkenstein, Daniel H. *Medical Students, Medical Schools and Society during Five Eras: Factors Affecting the Career Choices of Physicians 1958–1976*. Cambridge, Mass.: Ballinger, 1978.

Geiger, Roger L. *To Advance Knowledge: The Growth of American Research Universities, 1900–1940*. New York: Oxford University Press, 1986.

Gill, Gordon N. "The End of the Physician-Scientist?" *American Scholar*. 53 (1984): 353–368.

Gouldner, Alvin W. "Cosmopolitans and Locals: Toward an Analysis of Latent Social Roles." *Administrative Science Quarterly*. 2 (1957): 281–306.

Graham, John B. "Recruiting of Faculty." *North Carolina Medical Journal*. 47 (March 1986): 145–146.

Halpern, Sydney A. *American Pediatrics*. Berkeley: University of California Press, 1988.

______. "Professional Schools in the American University." In *The Academic Profession: National, Disciplinary, and Institutional Settings*, ed. Burton R. Clark. Berkeley: University of California Press, 1987.

Herman, Samuel S., and Allen M. Singer. "Basic Scientists in Clinical Departments of Medical Schools." *Clinical Research.* 34 (April 1986): 149–158.

Hilles, William C., Gerlandino Agro, Joseph Rosenthal, and David Sinclair. *An In-Depth Study of Seven Medical Practice Plans: An Analysis of Their Evolution and Operations.* Washington, D.C.: Association of American Medical Colleges, 1977.

Hillman, Bruce J., Laurie L. Fajardo, Donald B. Witzke, Diego Cardenas, Mark Irion, and John V. Fulginiti. "Factors Influencing Radiologists to Choose Research Careers." *Investigative Radiology.* 24 (November 1989a): 842–848.

Hillman, Bruce J., Laurie L. Fajardo, Donald B. Witzke, Mark Irion, Diego Cardenas, and John V. Fulginiti. "Factors Influencing the Success of Academic Radiologists in Publishing Research." *Investigative Radiology.* 24 (November 1989b): 849–854.

Holloway, Richard L., Kathryn L. Hale, and Robert E. Rakel. "Academic Promotion and Tenure in U.S. Family Medicine Units." *Academic Medicine.* 64 (May 1989): 270–272.

Jolly, Paul. "Faculty Age Distribution and Research Productivity." Paper presented at the Annual Meeting of the Association of American Medical Colleges, New Orleans, La., 27 October 1986.

Jones, Robert F., Marcie Foster Mirsky, and Joseph A. Keyes, Jr. "Clinical Practice of Medical School Faculties: An AAMC Survey of Problems and Issues." *Journal of Medical Education.* 60 (December 1985): 897–910.

Josiah Macy Jr. Foundation. *Report of the Commission for the Study of the Governance of the Academic Medical Center.* New York: Josiah Macy Jr. Foundation, 1970.

Kinder, Barbara K. "Being an Academic Surgeon." *Connecticut Medicine.* 53 (September 1989): 525–527.

Lehman, Thomas J. A., Daniel B. Magilavy, and Robert Warren. "Pediatric Rheumatology Manpower and Training: Planning for the 1990s." Hospital for Special Surgery, New York, New York, 1989.

Lewis, Irving J., and Cecil G. Sheps. *The Sick Citadel.* Cambridge, Mass.: Oelgeschlager, Gunn & Hain, 1983.

Light, Donald W. "The Development of Professional Schools in America." In *The Transformation of Higher Learning 1860–1930,* ed. Konrad H. Jarausch. Chicago: University of Chicago Press, 1983.

Littlefield, John W. "On the Difficulty of Combining Basic Research and Patient Care." *American Journal of Human Genetics.* 36 (July 1984): 731–735.

McShane, Michael G. *Medical Schools in the United States.* Washington, D.C.: Association of American Medical Colleges, 1977.

National Research Council. *On the Status of Medical School Faculty and Clinical Research Manpower, 1968–1990*. Washington, D.C.: Association of American Medical Colleges, 1981.

Neinstein, Lawrence S., and Richard G. MacKenzie. "Prior Training and Recommendations for Future Training of Clinical Research Faculty Members." *Academic Medicine*. 64 (January 1989): 32–35.

Parris, Maureen, and Edward J. Stemmler. "Development of Clinician-Educator Faculty Track at the University of Pennsylvania." *Journal of Medical Education*. 59 (June 1984): 465–470.

Pearse, Warren H., Judy G. Fielden, and Donald M. Sherline. "Obstetric-Gynecologic Academic Manpower." *Obstetrics & Gynecology*. 70 (September 1987): 403–407.

Petersdorf, Robert G. "The Academic Mating Game." *New England Journal of Medicine*. 298 (1 June 1978a): 1290–1294.

______. "The Doctors' Dilemma." *New England Journal of Medicine*. 299 (21 September 1978b): 628–634.

Pritchett, Edward L. C., Galen S. Wagner, Andrew G. Wallace, and Joseph C. Greenfield. "Career Choices of 135 Cardiology Trainees at Duke University Medical Center from 1970 to 1984." *American Journal of Cardiology*. 57 (1 February 1986): 313–315.

Schofield, J. R. *New and Expanded Medical Schools, Mid-Century to the 1980s*. San Francisco: Jossey-Bass, 1984.

Shattuck, Frederick C., and J. Lewis Bremer. "The Medical School." In *The Development of Harvard University*, ed. Samuel Eliot Morison. Cambridge: Harvard University Press, 1930.

Sherman, Charles R., and Terry Bryll. "Educational Origins of M.D. Faculty Members in Five Groups of Medical Schools." *Journal of Medical Education*. 57 (September 1982): 659–665.

Smith, Roger D., Robert E. Anderson, and Ellis S. Benson. "Manpower Needs and Supply in Academic Pathology." *Archives of Pathology and Laboratory Medicine*. 109 (October 1985): 889–893.

______. "Some Characteristics of Academic Departments of Pathology in the United States." *Archives of Pathology and Laboratory Medicine*. 111 (April 1987): 393–396.

Starr, Paul. *The Social Transformation of American Medicine*. New York: Basic Books, 1982.

Stevens, Rosemary. *American Medicine and the Public Interest*. New Haven, Conn.: Yale University Press, 1971.

______. "Graduate Medical Education: A Continuing History." *Journal of Medical Education*. 53 (January 1978): 1–18.

Stossel, Thomas P. "Brave New Medicine." *Journal of Clinical Investigation*. 80 (October 1987): 921–927.

Swanson, August G. "Medical Education in the United States and Canada." *Journal of Medical Education*. 59 (November 1984): 35–56.

Vevier, Charles, ed. *Flexner: 75 Years Later*. Lanham, Md.: University Press of America, 1987.

Weil, Peter A., and Mary Kay Schleiter. "National Study of Internal Medicine Manpower: VI. Factors Predicting Preferences of Residents for Careers in Primary Care or Subspecialty Care and Clinical Practice or Academic Medicine." *Annals of Internal Medicine*. 94 (May 1981): 691–703.

Worrell, John A., Alan C. Winfield, Frank E. Carroll, Jr., Faxon Payne, and John H. Beveridge. "Returning to Academic Radiology: Why Am I Doing This?" *Radiology*. 172 (September 1989): 874.

Wyngaarden, James B. "The Clinical Investigator as an Endangered Species." *New England Journal of Medicine*. 301 (6 December 1979): 1254–1259.

Zimny, George H., and Lindbergh S. Sata. "Influence of Factors Before and During Medical School on Choice of Psychiatry as a Specialty." *American Journal of Psychiatry*. 143 (January 1986): 77–80.

Index

About the Author

DOLORES L. BURKE is Special Assistant to the President of Duke University. She has published numerous articles on the academic job market and is the author of *A New Academic Marketplace* (Greenwood, 1988).